Work Stress Induced Chronic Diseases in Construction

This book aims to fill a gap in the current construction health and safety research and discover new knowledge about work stress induced chronic diseases among construction industry professionals. In achieving these aims, the book investigates:

- the nature and extent of psychosocial stressors experienced by construction professionals, stress management tactics applied and the impact on mental health
- the prevalence and occurrence patterns of serious chronic conditions such as insomnia, obesity, musculoskeletal disorders and vision impairment
- aetiological pathways from job stressors through chronic diseases to job performance.

While there are many studies, policies and regulations aiming to look after the health of construction workers, little attention is paid to construction professionals. By applying advanced analytical methods to data collected in a national survey of construction professionals in Australia, the author presents new scientific evidence which can be used to help establish equitable workers' compensation treatments and outcomes for construction professionals in line with other professions. Moreover, the research and analysis are underpinned by theories and literature from public health and epidemiological disciplines in addition to literature from construction, and work health, safety and wellbeing domains. It is essential reading for any health policy makers and researchers in the fields of health and safety and construction management.

Imriyas Kamardeen is Professor of Construction Management in the School of Architecture and Built Environment at Deakin University, Australia.

Spon Research

Publishes a stream of advanced books for built environment researchers and professionals from one of the world's leading publishers. The ISSN for the Spon Research programme is ISSN 1940-7653 and the ISSN for the Spon Research E-book programme is ISSN 1940-8005

Work Stress Induced Chronic Diseases in Construction

Discoveries Using Data Analytics

Imriyas Kamardeen

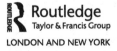

Routledge
Taylor & Francis Group

LONDON AND NEW YORK

First published 2021
by Routledge
2 Park Square, Milton Park, Abingdon, Oxon OX14 4RN

and by Routledge
52 Vanderbilt Avenue, New York, NY 10017

Routledge is an imprint of the Taylor & Francis Group, an informa business

© 2021 Imriyas Kamardeen

British Library Cataloguing-in-Publication Data
A catalogue record for this book is available from the British Library

Library of Congress Cataloging-in-Publication Data
Names: Kamardeen, Imriyas, author.
Title: Work stress induced chronic diseases in construction :
discoveries using data analytics / Imriyas Kamardeen.
Description: 1. | Boca Raton : CRC Press, 2021. |
Series: Spon research | Includes index.
Identifiers: LCCN 2020046260 (print) | LCCN 2020046261 (ebook) |
ISBN 9780367631147 (hardback) | ISBN 9781003118725 (ebook)
Subjects: LCSH: Medicine, Psychosomatic. | Stress (Physiology) |
Construction workers–Health and hygiene.
Classification: LCC RC49 .K33 2021 (print) |
LCC RC49 (ebook) | DDC 616.08–dc23
LC record available at https://lccn.loc.gov/2020046260
LC ebook record available at https://lccn.loc.gov/2020046261

ISBN: 978-0-367-63114-7 (hbk)
ISBN: 978-0-367-63302-8 (pbk)
ISBN: 978-1-003-11872-5 (ebk)

Typeset in Baskerville
by Newgen Publishing UK

Dedicated to my parents, my wife Zakia and my children Mahdiyya, Imaad and Haadi

Contents

Figures

Tables

Preface

Medical science warns that enduring excessive stress for a long period can cause serious chronic diseases, which could eventually lead to early mortality. Further evidence from the public health domain reveals that suffering chronic diseases is positively associated with increased depressive symptoms. Recent research globally concluded that the construction industry professionals endure excessive work stress. All the evidence collectively argues that construction professionals, due to enduring excessive work stress, are at high risk of suffering a vicious cycle between chronic diseases and depression, slowly resulting in the worse form of disability that could cripple not only individuals but also their families. Furthermore, this has been found to be a key contributor of suicide in Australia.

Despite its importance, the relationship between work stress and the development of chronic diseases among construction professionals is largely unexplored. Most of the existing work on work stress among construction professionals only discusses the causes of work stress, stress moderators, stress coping methods and the effects of stress on psychological health and job performance. This book addresses this important gap, discovering new knowledge and practical insights, by applying data analytics methods on data collected in a national survey in Australia.

The book exists in the intersection of four main bodies of knowledge such as construction management, work health and safety, occupational psychology and epidemiology. Yet, the book is presented in a very accessible way so that it will benefit practitioners, researchers and tertiary students alike. The chapters of the book discuss findings of different but connected recent research studies that use various data analytics techniques to derive models and insights for multiple types of audiences. The salient features of the book that make it relevant to the different audiences are as follows:

- It demonstrates how construction organisations may utilise contemporary research and theories to improve psychosocial conditions at work that compromise sustainable business performance.
- It is practical and value adding to the construction industry internationally.
- It presents clear and easy-to-follow explanations to organisations in the construction industry, WHS professionals, medical/clinical practitioners, insurance providers, researchers and tertiary students on: (1) the health

consequences of work stress; (2) analytical processes for discovering know-ledge on complex causalities; and (3) causal models.
- It can be a key reference material for human resources divisions of organisations, WHS practitioners and authorities, researchers and students.
- It enhances the body of knowledge in construction WHS, leveraged by theories from the epidemiological and occupational psychology fields.
- As far as the author is aware, no book has been written on work stress induced chronic diseases in construction, as this book does. It would be the first book ever published internationally.

In brief, although the book is research-based, it is significantly geared towards equally improving industry practices, education and research.

Disclaimer

Whilst the author has taken reasonable care in the preparation of this book, the use of the book is at your own risk and on an 'as is' basis. The author makes no expressed or implied warranty of any kind and will not be liable to you for any errors or omissions.

The author excludes any liability to you or anyone claiming through you for any loss, liability or damage whether direct or indirect suffered or incurred by you or a third party arising from or in connection with the use of the book, including any information derived from it.

You should carefully review any recommendations or information contained in this book and obtain independent verification from a suitably qualified professional before acting on any of those recommendations. No responsibility is assumed by the author for any injury and/or damage to a person or property arising from any methods, instructions or recommendations contained in this book.

Acknowledgements

I am morally obliged to express my gratitude to various individuals and organisations for their invaluable support that allowed me to make this book a success.

First and foremost, I sincerely thank the almighty God for giving me the ability in every dimension to author this book.

I would like to thank my employer, Deakin University Australia, for providing me with the necessary resources and support for completing this book.

I am grateful to the professional institutions that helped me circulate an online survey to their members to collect primary data required for the research that underpins the chapters of the book. The professional institutions include the Australian Institute of Architects (AIA), Australian Institute of Building (AIB), Australian Institute of Building Surveyors (AIBS), Australian Institute of Health and Safety (AIHS), Australian Institute of Quantity Surveyors (AIQS), Facilities Management Association of Australia (FMA), Chartered Institute of Building (CIOB) – Australian Chapter, Royal Institution of Charters Surveyors (RICS) – Oceania Chapter, Master Builders Association of Victoria and the Civil Contractors Federation. Likewise, I would like to thank the Australian construction industry professionals who responded to the survey. The book would not have been possible without their support.

Special thanks go to Göran Runeson for providing feedback on the chapters of the book, which helped me improve their readability.

I would like to extend my appreciation to my wife, Zakia Rizvi, for her love, patience and continued support to my career, especially during the development of this book, and to my children, Mahdiyya, Imaad and Haadi, for their love that rejuvenates me regularly to keep going.

Last but not least, I would like to thank my parents, extended family, friends and colleagues for their encouragement and support of different forms during my academic career, particularly during the development of this book.

Abbreviations

ANOVA	Analysis of variance
BMI	Body mass index
CBT-I	Cognitive behaviour therapy for insomnia
CFI	Comparative fit index
CHAID	Chi-squared automatic interaction detection
CRT	Classification and regression tree
CVDs	Cardiovascular disorders
ERI	Effort-reward imbalance
GFI	Goodness-of-fit index
HPA	Hypothalamic-pituitary-adrenal
HSE	Health and safety executive
IoT	Internet of Things
MDS	Multidimensional scaling
MSDs	Musculoskeletal disorders
NFI	Normed fit index
PTSD	Post-traumatic stress disorder
QUEST	Quick, Unbiased, Efficient Statistical Tree
RMSEA	Root mean square error of approximation
TLI	Tucker-Lewis index
UK	United Kingdom
US	United States
WHO	World Health Organization
WHS	Work health and safety
WLC	Work–life conflict
WMSDs	Work-related musculoskeletal disorders

1 Introduction

Acceptable work health, safety and wellbeing of the workforce is a critical aspect for the social sustainability of any nation. This is also essential for the economic sustainability of employees, employers and the society. Whilst the exposure to traditional hazards on construction sites has declined due to the advent of innovative technologies and improved work policies and procedures, particularly in developed countries, the health and wellbeing of employees are threatened by stressful psychosocial work environments (Siegrist and Li 2018). The construction industry is particularly notorious for psychosocial stressors globally and as such its professionals endure excessive work stress (Chan, Nwaogu and Naslund 2020; Bowen et al. 2018; Sunindijo and Kamardeen 2017; Bowen et al. 2014; Leung, Chan and Dongyu 2011; Love, Edwards and Irani 2010; Campbell 2006).

Effects of work stress on construction professionals

Enduring work stress for an extended period could lead to more serious outcomes for employees and organisations. Work stress effects on employees undermine the social sustainability whereby employees are adversely affected in three dimensions such as mental wellbeing, physical health and job performance. Lupien et al. (2009) argued that chronic stress triggers the presence of high levels of glucocorticoids, which affects the frontal cortex and hippocampus of the brain, increasing the risk of depressive disorders. Work stress has also been found to cause anxiety disorders (Melchior et al. 2007). To evidence this, Campbell (2006) reported that approximately 70% of construction professionals were inflicted with anxiety and/or depression as a direct result of experiencing excessive work stress. Dollard (2001) warned that long-term psychological effects of work stress may result in permanent mental illnesses and/or even suicide. Moreover, public health literature claims that enduring long-term excessive stress can cause chronic and serious diseases, such as obesity, hyperlipidaemia, type 2 diabetes, high cholesterol levels, coronary heart disease, cardiovascular disorders, musculoskeletal pains, gastrointestinal problems, headache and migraine, prolonged fatigue, respiratory infections, reproductive system disorders, immune system weakening and early mortality (Salvagioni et al. 2017). Further evidence from the public health domain revealed a bi-directional relationship that suffering chronic diseases such as arthritis, lung disease, cardiac disease and cancer were positively associated with increased depressive symptoms over time (Bisschop et al. 2004).

It is derived from this that stressed out employees are at high risk of suffering a vicious cycle between chronic diseases and mental ill-health, slowly resulting in the worse form of disability that could cripple not only individuals but also the socio-economic status and the livelihood of their families. Moreover, the combination of mental and physical illnesses can adversely impact on an employee's work performance and potential. When a large number of employees suffer the previously mentioned consequences, it will significantly impact on organisational operations via increased absenteeism, presenteeism, low productivity, poor work safety records, high insurance and compensation costs, high employee turnover, continual recruitment and training costs, low job satisfaction, industrial actions and reputation damage. These would impact on the economic sustainability of construction organisations (Kamardeen 2019).

The multifaceted impacts discussed in the preceding paragraphs could collectively cause enormous socio-economic losses for affected employees, their families, businesses and society broadly. Examples of possible economic losses for individual employees are loss of salaries, reduction of professional capacities and increased medical costs. Social costs include pain and suffering, strain on relationships, lifestyle changes, lowered self-esteem and burden on family (European Union 2011). When the socio-economic costs suffered by all affected employees are aggregated, they can constitute a huge loss to the society in the form of production loss, increased welfare and medical costs, diminished standard of living and reductions in human labour potential (European Union 2011). Safe Work Australia, for example, estimated that Australia loses $10.9 billion yearly due to lost productivity resulting from work-related mental stress that significantly impacts on workers' health and performance (Safe Work Australia 2018). The work-related mental disorder profile produced by Safe Work Australia ascertained that about 7,800 Australians receive compensation for work-related mental stress annually (Safe Work Australia 2015). An Australian study conducted in 2016 estimated that nearly 75% of employees experienced stress at work in 2015 (Phillip 2019). Furthermore, a steep rise in suicide, substance abuse and serious illnesses such as cardiovascular disorders, tumour, cancer, diabetes and obesity have been identified as the most prevalent consequences of work stress in Australia (Roche et al. 2012; Waters 2017). Similar statistics and conditions are prevalent elsewhere in other countries too.

Current knowledge

Several studies on work stress in the construction industry have been conducted to date by many researchers around the world, resulting in numerous publications, particularly journal articles on this theme. Most of these studies focussed on construction professionals and can be grouped into three categories.

The first group of studies focussed on the causes and psychological consequences of work stress in construction. Sunindijo and Kamardeen (2017) investigated the psychosocial stressors endured by construction professionals in Australia and their impacts on stress, anxiety and depression experiences. They further assessed whether women professionals in the construction industry differed from their men colleagues in their exposure and experiences. Bowen, Govender and Edwards (2014) investigated how job demand, job control, work–life imbalance and workplace support impacted on construction professionals' experiences of stress in South Africa. In a subsequent study, Bowen, Govender and Edwards (2014) explored occupational stress-related predictors of psychological, physiological and sociological strain effects among construction professionals in South Africa. Recently, Bowen et al. (2018) examined the relationship between work contact, work–family conflict and consequent outcomes of psychological distress and sleep problems experienced by South African construction professionals. Similarly, Leung, Chan and Yu (2009) modelled the causal relationship between workplace stressors and stress of construction project managers in Hong Kong.

The second set of research explored moderators of work stress and the effects of stress coping methods and social support at work on psychological outcomes. Kamardeen and Sunindijo (2017) studied the influence of personal characteristics and argued that individual differences in personality traits can result in different stress outcomes for two different professionals who experience the same psychosocial conditions at work. Love, Edwards and Irani (2010) compared the nature of self-stress and mental health, and the effect of social support between construction professionals who work on site and in office environments in Australia. Lingard and Francis (2006) examined the effect of perceived organisational support and support from supervisors and co-workers in the relationship between work–family conflict and burnout of construction professionals and managers in Australia. Haynes and Love (2004) investigated how coping and affect (both negative and positive) influence adjustment (anxiety, depression and stress) among male construction project managers in Australia.

The third category of research on this theme examined the effect of work stress on job performance. Leung, Liu and Wong (2006) studied the impact of stress coping behaviour on estimating accuracy of quantity surveyors/estimators in Hong Kong. Leung, Chan and Dongyu (2011) examined the structural linear relationship between job stress, burnout, psychological stress and performance among construction project managers in Hong Kong.

In summary, the causes of work stress in construction professionals, stress moderators, stress coping and the effects of stress on psychological health and job performance have been explored quite well in the last two decades, resulting in a modest level of knowledge on the theme.

Focus of the book

Despite the recognition that work stress is a risk factor for serious chronic diseases such as cardiovascular disorders, type 2 diabetes, obesity, musculoskeletal disorders, gastrointestinal problems, respiratory infections, reproductive system disorders, immune system weakening and early mortality (Salvagioni et al. 2017), there has been very little research on the relationship between work stress and the development of chronic diseases among construction professionals. Lack of scientific evidence on the health sufferings endured by construction professionals may disadvantage them immensely. For instance, existing workers' compensation systems do not consider work stress as compensable unless it leads to reportable psychological disorders. Similarly, work stress as an occupational cause for the previously mentioned chronic diseases must be well-established to qualify for any workers' compensation. While there have been many work health policies, and regulations to care for the health of operatives, little attention is paid to construction professionals. Scientific evidence needs to be established to support equitable workers' compensation treatments and outcomes for construction professionals too.

In light of the research gap identified, this book aims to discover new knowledge about work stress induced chronic diseases among construction industry professionals. In achieving the aim, the book investigates:

- the nature and extent of psychosocial stressors experienced by construction professionals, stress management tactics applied and the impact on mental health
- the prevalence and occurrence patterns of work stress induced chronic diseases among construction professionals
- aetiological pathways from job stressors through chronic diseases to job performance.

Research methodology

The research that underpinned the development of this book adopted the positivistic paradigm broadly. The discovery of new knowledge that is discussed within each chapter was achieved by applying different analytics methods on data collected in a national survey of construction professionals in Australia. Moreover, the research and analysis were reinforced by theories and literature from public health and epidemiological disciplines in addition to literature from construction, and work health, safety and wellbeing domains.

Survey

A questionnaire survey approach was adopted for primary data collection. As demonstrated by Table 1.1, the questionnaire had eight sections, namely respondent's background, job stressors, work–private life conflict, chronic job stress, stress coping methods, mental health effects, physical health effects, job outcomes and organisational interventions. A 4-point Likert scale was used to collect responses for the different sections, except for the respondent's background section, which used categorical responses. A copy of the full questionnaire is available in the Appendix.

Table 1.1 Sections of the questionnaire

Section	Response options

Respondent's background
1. Gender (male, female or other)
2. Age (≤20, 21–30, 31–40, 41–50, 51–60 or >60)
3. Marital status (married/de-facto, single or divorced/separated/widowed)
4. Organisation type (property development, PM, architecture, engineering, QS, builder, subcontractor, FM or other)
5. Organisation size (measured by # of full-time employees) (≤4, 5–19, 20–199 or ≥200)
6. Job title (text responses were received but categorised as junior professional, mid-career professional, senior professional or executive)
7. Experience (<1 year, 1–5 years, 6–10 years or >10 years)
8. Nature of employment (permanent, fixed-term contract or casual)
9. Hours worked weekly (<20, 20–30, 30–40, 40–50 or >50)
10. Workplace environment (site or office)
11. Income (<$40k, $40–60k, $60-80k, $80–100k, $100–120k, $120–150k or >$150k)

Job stressors
In the past 6 months at work how often did you experience:
1. Poor/dangerous work environment
2. Excessive workload
3. Unpredictable work hours
4. Time pressure
5. Job autonomy
6. Job appropriateness
7. Flexibility
8. Supportive feedback
9. Line manager support
10. Co-worker support
11. Harassment
12. Bullying
13. Discrimination
14. Role ambiguity
15. Adequate job resources
16. Staff consultation
17. Sufficient remuneration
18. Reward
19. Job security
20. Career prospect

Measured using the scale of:
• Never
• Sometimes
• Often
• Always

Work–private life conflict
In the past 6 months how often did you experience:
1. Lack of energy for private life
2. Lack of time for private life
3. Family complained about too much work
4. Other personal life stressors

Measured using the scale of:
• Never
• Sometimes
• Often
• Always

(continued)

Table 1.1 Cont.

Section	Response options

Chronic job stress
In the past 4 weeks how often did you experience:
  1. Poor sleep
  2. Restlessness
  3. Irritability
  4. Tensed
  5. Nervousness

Measured using the scale of:
• Never
• Sometimes
• Often
• Always

Stress coping methods
In the past 4 weeks how often did you engage in the following stress coping methods:
  1. Problem-solving
  2. Positive reappraisal
  3. Seeking support
  4. Relaxation
  5. Physical activity
  6. Leisure and humour
  7. Eating balanced diet
  8. Adequate sleep
  9. Isolation
  10. Alcohol/drug use
  11. Smoking
  12. Emotional eating
  13. Criticise/blame others
  14. Compulsive spending
  15. Denial/ignoring as if nothing happened
  16. Releasing tension

Measured using the scale of:
• Not at all
• Several days
• More than half the days
• Nearly every day

Physical and mental health effects
A) In the past 6 months how often were you bothered by/treated for:
  1. High blood pressure
  2. High cholesterol
  3. High blood sugar level
  4. Angina
  5. Heart muscle weakening
  6. Heart attack
  7. Stroke
  8. Diabetes
  9. Weight gain/obesity
  10. Gastrointestinal disorders
  11. Asthma
  12. Bronchitis
  13. Pneumonia
  14. Eczema
  15. Chronic headache/migraine
  16. Insomnia
  17. Back, neck or shoulder pain
  18. Arthritis
  19. Blurred eye vision
  20. Slow healing

Measured using the scale of:
• Never
• Once or twice
• Monthly
• Weekly

Table 1.1 Cont.

Section	Response options
21. Sexual dysfunction 22. Reproductive system disorder 23. Burnout 24. Anxiety 25. Depression	
B) Do you believe that job stress may have caused this illness? (this was asked for each heath problem above)	Dichotomous response –Yes / No
Organisational interventions In the past 6 months how often did your organisation apply the following interventions to improve employee wellbeing: 1. Improving work policies and conditions 2. Changing working conditions and practices 3. Skill improvement for employees 4. Training managers on employee wellbeing 5. Stress management training for employees 6. Facilitating relaxation and exercise programs 7. Promoting peer support 8. Psychological counselling, care & therapy 9. Rehabilitation & RTW for wellbeing issues	Measured using the scale of: • Never • Sometimes • Often • Always
Job outcomes In the past 6 months how would you rate your: 1. Job satisfaction 2. Job performance	Measured using a scale of 1 (low) to 10 (high)

Study sample

The population for the study was professionals in the Australian AEC industry, which include architects, engineers, project managers, construction managers, site managers, quantity surveyors/cost managers, building surveyors, facilities managers, contract administrators, builders, subcontractors, etc. It was essential to determine an appropriate sample size and a sampling method for the survey. The determination of the sample size for a survey that collects responses on a Likert-scale is different from other types of study that collect continuous or binary responses. Park and Jung (2009) proposed a formula for determining sample sizes for Likert scale-based surveys and they derived tables thereof to simplify the sample size computation. Table 1.2 shows the most applicable and recommended table by them for use when a 4-point or 5-point Likert scale is used. K in the table refers to the number of points in the Likert scale and D is the expected confidence level. The present study used a 4-point Likert scale, except for two variables that used a 10-point scale. Hence, a sample size of 241 would be sufficient to achieve a confidence level of 5%, based on Table 1.2.

Table 1.2 Sample size formula for Likert scale-based surveys

K \ D	1%	2%	3%	4%	5%	10%
1	9,604	2,401	1,068	601	385	97
2	7,203	1,801	801	451	289	73
3	6,403	1,601	712	401	257	65
4	6,003	1,501	667	376	241	61
5	5,763	1,441	641	361	231	58
6	5,603	1,401	623	351	225	57
7	5,488	1,372	610	343	220	55
8	5,403	1,351	601	338	217	55
9	5,336	1,334	593	334	214	54
10	5,283	1,321	587	331	212	53

Following the random sampling principle, an online questionnaire survey was conducted from October 2019 to February 2020, inclusive, with AEC professionals who work in major cities of Australia. They were approached through professional institutions such as the Australian Institute of Architects (AIA), Australian Institute of Building (AIB), Australian Institute of Building Surveyors (AIBS), Australian Institute of Health and Safety (AIHS), Australian Institute of Quantity Surveyors (AIQS), Facilities Management Association of Australia (FMA), Chartered Institute of Building (CIOB) – Australian Chapter, Royal Institution of Charters Surveyors (RICS) – Oceania Chapter, Master Builders Association of Victoria and Civil Contractors Federation. Additionally, requests were sent to the professional connections of the author who were attached to various organisations in the AEC industry. A total of 310 construction professionals completed the survey. Of the 310 respondents, 63 had not completed the questionnaire fully and therefore were removed, resulting in 247 usable responses.

Respondents

Table 1.3 presents the complete socio-demographic characteristics of the respondents of the usable responses. More than 75% of them were male, which is symbolic of the male dominated characteristics of the construction industry. However, the representation of females in the survey (21%) was almost double the industry representation of 11% (Turnbull 2016). The age group of 20 to 30 accounted for almost one-third whilst groups 31 to 40 and 41 to 50 represented almost equally at around a quarter each. In brief, around 80% of the respondents fell in the age range of 20 to 50. In terms of marital status, two-thirds of them were in a married/de-facto relationship while a small fraction (7%) were separated/divorced/widowed. One-fourth of them were single. This relationship status could play a role in work–life conflict and stress coping, and therefore is an important factor to note (Sunindijo and Kamardeen 2017). About half of the respondents had a moderate level of work experience of 1 to 5 years. Similarly, junior and mid-career professionals accounted for nearly one-fourth

Table 1.3 Respondents' profiles

Respondent characteristic	Number	Percent
Gender:		
• Male	192	77.7
• Female	52	21.1
• Other	3	1.2
Age:		
• Below 20	1	.4
• 20 to 30	75	30.4
• 31 to 40	59	23.9
• 41 to 50	60	24.3
• 51 to 60	32	13.0
• Over 60	19	7.7
• Unspecified	1	.4
Marital status:		
• Married/de-facto	166	67.2
• Single, never married	63	25.5
• Single, separated/divorced/widowed	17	6.8
• Unspecified	1	.4
Organisation type:		
• Property developer	12	4.9
• PM consultancy	20	8.1
• Architectural consultancy	23	9.3
• Engineering consultancy	19	7.7
• QS consultancy	41	16.6
• Builder (main)	79	32.0
• Subcontractor	19	7.7
• Facility manager	5	2.0
• Other	29	11.7
Organisation size:		
• 4 or less employees	22	8.9
• 5 to 19 employees	45	18.2
• 20 to 199 employees	78	31.6
• 200 or more employees	101	58.9
• Unknown	1	.4
Experience:		
• Less than 1 year	29	11.7
• 1 to 5 years	118	47.8
• 6 to 10 years	37	15.0
• Over 10 years	62	25.1
Occupation level:		
• Junior professionals	66	26.7
• Mid-career professional	57	23.1
• Senior professional	79	32.0
• Executives	39	15.8
• Unspecified	6	2.4
Workplace environment:		
• Office	202	81.8
• Site	45	18.2

(continued)

Table 1.3 Cont.

Respondent characteristic	Number	Percent
Annual salary:		
• Less than $40k	8	3.2
• $40k to $60k	19	7.7
• $60 to $80k	29	11.7
• $80 to $100k	38	15.4
• $100k to $120k	27	10.9
• $120k to $150k	43	17.4
• Over $150k	78	31.6
• Unspecified	5	2.0

each, making a total of half the respondents and corresponding to the fraction for experience level of 1 to 5 years. Senior professionals who are with senior management positions represented almost one-third and executives constituted one-sixth. Moreover, around one-third of them were employees of main builders, followed by a proportion of one-sixth from QS consultancies. Although around one-third were builders, only half of them were working predominantly on construction sites. More than half of the respondents were employed at large organisations and around the same proportion of them received an annual income of above $100k with one-third of all receiving over $150k. This suggests that the construction professionals surveyed were well-paid in Australia.

Pilot screening

The textual Likert scales used in the survey were assigned numerical codes in the following manner to enable quantitative analysis and uniformity in the way measurement scales of data are presented:

- Scale 1: never = 0, sometimes = 1, often = 2, always = 3.
- Scale 2: not satisfied = 0, somewhat satisfied = 1, satisfied = 2, very satisfied = 3.
- Scale 3: never = 0, once or twice = 1, monthly = 2, weekly = 3.
- Scale 4: not at all = 0, several days = 1, more than half the days = 2, nearly every day = 3.

Subsequently, a pilot analysis was carried out to understand the prevalence of different diseases among construction professionals. The survey had included 22 physical and three psychological health effects due to work stress. Participants' responses to the following question were analysed:

- In the past 6 months how often were you bothered by/treated for:
  1. High blood pressure
  2. High cholesterol

3. High blood sugar level
4. Angina
5. Heart muscle weakening
6. Heart attack
7. Stroke
8. Diabetes
9. Obesity/weight gain
10. Gastrointestinal disorders
11. Asthma
12. Bronchitis
13. Pneumonia
14. Eczema
15. Chronic headache/migraine
16. Insomnia
17. Back, neck & shoulder pain
18. Arthritis
19. Blurred eye vision
20. Slow healing
21. Sexual dysfunction
22. Reproductive system disorder
23. Burnout
24. Anxiety
25. Depression

The prevalence and severity levels of the diseases were combinedly gauged using the means and standard deviations of the responses received and Table 1.4 summarises the results. It is evident that the following conditions are more prevalent among construction professionals out of the 25 diseases/disorders assessed:

- musculoskeletal pains
- psychological disorders
- insomnia
- weight gain/obesity
- blurred eye vision.

Literature on occupational psychology strongly suggests that cardiovascular disorders are natural physical health consequences of work stress. However, the findings here did not reveal a strong prevalence of these diseases. Hence, the book focusses on the five chronic conditions previously listed.

Table 1.4 Pilot screening of disease prevalence

Disease	Mean	Std. Deviation
Back, neck or shoulder pain	1.07	1.077
Anxiety	1.03	1.094
Depression	.81	1.027
Insomnia	.79	1.118
Weight gain/Obesity	.77	0.986
Burnout	.77	1.035
Blurred eye vision	.54	.907
Migraine or chronic headache	.48	.854
Gastrointestinal disorders	.44	.855
Eczema	.42	.865
High blood pressure	.39	.798
High cholesterol	.36	.777
Sexual dysfunction	.30	.729
Angina	.26	.646
Arthritis	.25	.693
High blood sugar level	.22	.600
Weakened immune system/slow healing	.17	.495
Asthma	.15	.517
Heart muscle weakening	.14	.520
Reproductive system disorders	.13	.511
Diabetes type 2	.09	.402
Bronchitis	.08	.365
Heart attack	.05	.283
Stroke	.04	.268
Pneumonia	.03	.195

Structure of the book

The book comprises seven chapters, and the contents of each chapter are outlined as follows.

Chapter 1: Introduction

This introductory chapter established the key arguments and themes that propel the book and provides a broad context for the remaining chapters in the book.

Chapter 2: Work stress induced psychological disorders in construction

The construction sector is regarded as a high-risk industry for work stress due to the inherent nature of its operations and work culture. Construction projects are generally characterised by complexity of parallel tasks/trades, tight time and cost constraints, uncertainty, complex multi-layered contractual relationships among various organisations, inter-personal conflicts, contractual disputes, excessive compliant and approval requirements, long work hours and poor physical work environments. Stress has become a general phenomenon for construction professionals because of dealing with these issues regularly in their projects, with reports claiming nearly 70% of them are suffering from anxiety and/or depression. This chapter aims to:

- explore psychosocial job stressors, work stress and psychological disorders endured by construction professionals and analyse how these vary across different professional groups, demographics, and sizes and types of organisations
- investigate the methods of work stress management deployed by individuals as well as construction organisations
- examine the interaction among stressors, work stress and stress management methods in producing mental health conditions among construction professionals.

Chapter 3: Work stress induced chronic insomnia in construction

Adequate, quality sleep is an essential human need that provides natural restoration for the central nervous and the physiological systems of the body. It directly affects the mental and physical health and performance, including brain and heart health, immune system, metabolism, emotional balance, productivity, attention, memory, learning, creativity and vitality. Recent epidemiological research revealed that sleep quality and quantity has been declining and the symptoms of insomnia have become more rampant among the working population due to work stress. It further claimed a reciprocal relationship between work stress and sleep, forming a vicious cycle, i.e. work stress affects an individual's sleep which in turn affects work performance, leading to more work stress.

This chapter investigates the prevalence of work stress induced chronic insomnia among construction professionals, and develops a causal model connecting psychosocial stressors at work, chronic insomnia and job performance. It further examines the influence of factors such as job role, gender and age on insomnia occurrences. Then, the chapter checks for evidence for the prevalence of an association between chronic insomnia and other medical complications in construction professionals. Finally, techniques for treating insomnia are discussed.

Chapter 4: Work stress induced musculoskeletal disorders in construction

Work-related musculoskeletal disorders (WMSDs) have traditionally been believed to be caused by physical forces or ergonomic conditions at work. In the construction industry, WMSDs have largely been associated with operatives because of the understanding that only they are involved in physically strenuous activities. To this end, most research studies of WMSDs have focussed on physical factors, ergonomics and operatives in the construction industry. However, recent research in the epidemiology claimed that psychosocial conditions at work and work stress play an important role in the development of WMSDs. Given that the construction industry is notorious for work stress and with the evidence that work stress is a key cause of WMSDs, it is likely that a large proportion of construction professionals are susceptible to WMSDs. Moreover, the workers' compensation system largely recognises exposure to physical risk factors only when assessing claims for WMSDs. This is owing to the wide availability and acceptance of well-established epidemiological evidence. It is therefore paramount that a similar level of evidence is produced to lobby for the recognition of work stress induced WMSDs too in the workers' compensation system. To that end, this chapter explores the prevalence of work stress induced WMSDs among professionals in the Australian construction industry. It further develops a causal model connecting work stress, WMSDs and job performance outcomes.

Chapter 5: Work stress induced weight gain in construction

Public health literature argues that the primary cause of overweight and obesity is an imbalance between calories consumed and spent, which is a result of the combination of an increased consumption of calorie-dense food and decreased physical activity due to a sedentary lifestyle. Nonetheless, recently researchers have claimed that stress, including work stress, is a significant risk factor for overweight and obesity. Traditionally, obesity has not been considered as a WHS issue, but recent evidence shows strong associations between psychosocial work factors and obesity. Construction being notorious for work stress and poor psychosocial work environments, construction professionals may be at high risk of overweight and obesity and their subsequent complications. However, this is an unexplored topic in construction management literature. This chapter therefore investigates work stress induced weight gains among construction professionals. It further examines the influence of personal characteristics and individual stress coping methods on the association between work stress and overweight. Finally, the chapter assesses the association between weight gain and other health conditions among construction professionals.

Chapter 6: Work stress induced vision impairment in construction

World Health Organization (WHO) estimated that globally at least 2.2 billion people have a vision impairment. Eye health conditions such as uncorrected refractive errors, cataract, age-related macula degeneration, glaucoma, diabetic retinopathy, corneal opacity and trachoma are regarded as the immediate medical causes of vision impairment. Recent epidemiological studies have recognised that chronic mental stress and associated mental health conditions are significant risk factors for the development and progression of such eye health issues and thereby vision impairment. Workplace stress accounts for a significant portion of the mental health crisis in today's population. It can therefore be deduced that a significant portion of vision-related problems in the working population may be attributed to work stress. It is conclusive globally that professionals in the construction industry endure excessive work stress, suggesting that they are vulnerable to irreversible vision loss. However, this is thus far an underappreciated risk in construction health and safety literature. Hence, this chapter investigates work stress induced vision impairment among construction professionals. It examines the prevalence of vision loss, workplace psychosocial risk factors, stress coping methods that exacerbate vision loss, confounding factors that influence the relationship between work stress and vision impairment, and the impact on job outcomes.

Chapter 7: Concluding remarks

This final chapter brings together all the findings in the previous chapters into a coherent framework, and reports their practical implications for construction organisations, construction professionals, healthcare professionals, the workers' compensation scheme and policy makers. The chapter further discusses the potential use of the analytics methods applied in the book by other researchers and future research directions in the construction work health, safety and wellbeing theme.

References

Bisschop, M.I., Kriegsman, D.M., Beekman, A.T. and Deeg, D.J. (2004). Chronic diseases and depression: the modifying role of psychosocial resources. *Social Science & Medicine*, *59*(4), 721–733.

Bowen, P., Edwards, P., Lingard, H. and Cattell, K. (2014). Occupational stress and job demand, control and support factors among construction project consultants. *International Journal of Project Management*, *32*(7), 1273–1284.

Bowen, P., Govender, R. and Edwards, P. (2014). Structural equation modeling of occupational stress in the construction industry. *Journal of Construction Engineering and Management*, *140*(9), 04014042.

Bowen, P., Govender, R., Edwards, P. and Cattell, K. (2018). Work-related contact, work-family conflict, psychological distress and sleep problems experienced by construction professionals: an integrated explanatory model. *Construction Management and Economics*, *36*(3), 153–174.

Campbell, F. (2006). *Occupational Stress in the Construction Industry*. Ascot, UK: The Chartered Institute of Building.

Chan, A.P.C., Nwaogu, J.M. and Naslund, J.A. (2020). Mental ill-health risk factors in the construction industry: systematic review. *Journal of Construction Engineering and Management*, *146*(3), 04020004.

Dollard, M. (2001). Work stress theory and intervention: from evidence to policy a case study. In, *The NOHSC Symposium on the OHS Implications of Stress*.

European Union. (2011). Socio-economic costs of accidents at work and work-related ill health. Retrieved 13 April, 2016, from www.ilo.org/public/libdoc/igo/2011/468757.pdf.

Haynes, N.S. and Love, P.E.D. (2004). Psychological adjustment and coping among construction project managers. *Construction Management and Economics*, *22*(2), 129–140.

Kamardeen, I. (2019). *Preventing Workplace Incidents in Construction: Data Mining and Analytics Applications*. London: Routledge.

Kamardeen, I. and Sunindijo R.Y. (2017). Personal characteristics moderate work stress in construction professionals. *Journal of Construction Engineering and Management*, *143*(10). 1061/(ASCE)CO.1943-7862.0001386.

Leung, M., Chan, Y.S.I. and Dongyu, C. (2011). Structural linear relationships between job stress, burnout, physiological stress, and performance of construction project managers. *Engineering, Construction and Architectural Management, 18*(3), 312–328.

Leung, M.Y., Chan, Y.S. and Yu, J. (2009). Integrated model for the stressors and stresses of construction project managers in Hong Kong. *Journal of Construction Engineering and Management, 135*(2), 126–1344.

Leung, M.Y., Liu, A.M. and Wong, M.M.K. (2006). Impact of stress-coping behaviour on construction estimation performance. *Construction Management and Economics, 24*(1), 55–67.

Lingard, H. and Francis, V. (2006). Does a supportive work environment moderate the relationship between work-family conflict and burnout among construction professionals? *Construction Management and Economics, 24*(2), 185–196.

Love, P.E.D., Edwards, D.J. and Irani, Z. (2010). Work stress, support and mental health in construction. *Journal of Construction Engineering and Management, 136*(6), 650–658.

Lupien, S.J., McEwen, B.S., Gunnar, M.R. and Heim, C. (2009). Effects of stress throughout the lifespan on the brain, behaviour and cognition. *Nature Reviews Neuroscience, 10*(6), 434.

Melchior, M., Caspi, A., Milne, B.J., Danese, A., Poulton, R. and Moffitt, T.E. (2007). Work stress precipitates depression and anxiety in young, working women and men. *Psychological Medicine, 37*(8), 1119–1129.

Park, J. and Jung, M. (2009). A note on determination of sample size for a Likert scale. *Communications of the Korean Statistical Society, 16*(4), 669–673.

Phillip, K. (2019). Six ways your office can reduce stress. Retrieved 20 July, 2019, from www.morganlovell.co.uk/knowledge/opinion-pieces/six-ways-your-office-can-reduce-stress/.

Roche, A.M., Fischer, J., Pidd, K., Lee, N., Battams, S. and Nicholas, R. (2012). Workplace mental illness and substance use disorders in male-dominated industries: A Systematic Literature Review. Retrieved 20 July, 2019, from www.beyondblue.org.au/docs/default-source/research-project-files/bw0203.pdf?sfvrsn=e0fcbae9_2.

Salvagioni, D.A.J., Melanda, F.N., Mesas, A.E., González, A.D., Gabani, F.L. and de Andrade, S.M. (2017). Physical, psychological and occupational consequences of job burnout: A systematic review of prospective studies. *PLoS ONE, 12*(10), e0185781

Siegrist, J. and Li, J. (2018). Work stress and the development of chronic diseases. *International Journal of Environmental Research and Public Health, 15*, 536.

Sunindijo, R.Y. and Kamardeen, I. (2017). Work stress is a threat to gender diversity in the construction industry. *Journal of Construction Engineering and Management, 143*(10), 04017073.

Turnbull, M. (2016). Supporting women in building and construction. Prime Minister of Australia, Commonwealth of Australia, Dept. of Employment, Australian Government, Canberra, Australia.

Waters, S. (2017). Suicide voices: testimonies of trauma in the French workplace. *Medical humanities, 43*(1), 24–29.

Safe Work Australia. (2015). Work-related mental disorders profile 2015. Retrieved 3 August, 2020, from www.safeworkaustralia.gov.au/doc/work-related-mental-disorders-profile-2015.

Safe Work Australia. (2018). Supporting business to provide a mentally healthy workplace. Retrieved 20 July, 2019, from www.safeworkaustralia.gov.au/book/supporting-business-provide-mentally-healthy-workplace.

2 Work stress induced psychological disorders in construction

Employment is an important aspect for the quality of life and being unemployed is a high-risk factor for mental disorders (Fryers, Melzer and Jenkins 2003). Despite the positive role of employment on one's living conditions, work stress caused by unpleasant physical and psychosocial workplaces are increasingly taxing the mental wellbeing of the working population around the world, affecting all industries and professions. For instance, work stress is the major cause of sickness absence in Great Britain and costs the economy over £5 billion a year (HSE 2019). Similarly, Safe Work Australia estimated that Australian businesses lose over $10 billion yearly due to lost productivity resulting from work-related mental stress that significantly impacts on workers' health and performance (Safe Work Australia 2018). Moreover, an Australian study conducted in 2016 estimated that nearly 75% of employees experienced stress at work in 2015 (Phillip 2019). Similarly, 83% of the US working population suffer from work stress and US businesses lose about $300 billion yearly due to work stress (The American Institute of Stress 2019).

Every industry and profession are represented in the statistics in the previous paragraph; some are more than the others. The construction sector is regarded as a high-risk industry for work stress due to the inherent nature of its operations and work culture. Construction projects are generally characterised by the parallel progress of complex tasks/trades, tight schedules and cost constraints, uncertainty, complex multi-layered contractual relationships among various organisations, inter-personal conflicts, contractual disputes, excessive compliant and approval requirements, long work hours and poor physical work environments (Bowen et al. 2018; Sunindijo and Kamardeen 2017). Stress has become a general phenomenon for construction professionals because of dealing with these issues regularly in their projects, with nearly 70% of them suffering from stress, anxiety or depression (CIOB 2006). This chapter aims to investigate:

- the psychosocial job stressors, work stress and mental ill-health endured by construction professionals and how these vary across different professional groups, demographics and sizes and types of organisations
- the methods of work stress management deployed by individuals as well as construction organisations

- causal pathways from stressors through work stress to psychological strains, along with the moderating effects of stress management methods.

The remainder of the chapter is arranged as follows. First, definitions and a model of work stress are established by drawing from occupational psychology literature to provide a robust framework to guide the investigation in the construction context. Then, the research and analysis methods deployed are explained. Following that the findings of the research are discussed in light of existing literature on work stress in construction. Finally, new insights for practical implications are drawn in the conclusion section.

Work stress

Stress is the psychological and physical state that results when one's resources are insufficient to cope with the demands and pressures of the situation (Michie 2002). Stress can emerge from any dimension of one's life. In the occupational context, work stress is experienced when one is confronted with poor physical and psychosocial conditions known as job stressors and s/he does not have adequate resources (i.e. skills, knowledge, time, support, decision latitude, traits, habits) to combat them (Levy 2010; Kamardeen 2020). The human body and mind respond to stress with symptoms, which can be categorised into four types:

- emotions – irritability, fatigue, anxiousness, worry, sadness
- behaviour – social withdrawal, aggression, unmotivated, eating and sleeping problems, tobacco/alcohol/drug use
- cognition – poor concentration and memory, poor organisation and decision making, errors, accidents
- physiology – palpitations, sweat, headache, nausea, somatic pains.

When stress is prolonged or too frequent (known as chronic stress), it makes changes in neuroendocrine, cardiovascular, autonomic and immunological functioning, leading to serious mental disorders and physical illnesses (Levy 2010; Landy and Conte 2006; Muchinsky 2006; Michie 2002).

Model of work stress

Many models of work stress have been proposed by occupational psychology theorists to date. Each model adopts a unique perspective in defining causes and consequences of work stress. The model shown in Figure 2.1 encapsulates the constructs postulated by existing theories and presents a holistic picture of the sources and outcomes of stress, along with stress moderators. As illustrated in the diagram, sources of stress at work, also referred to as job stressors, are categorised into multiple origins. Similarly, the consequences of enduring work stress are classified into three types of strain: psychological, physiological and occupational. Several other factors can interact on the etiological pathway between

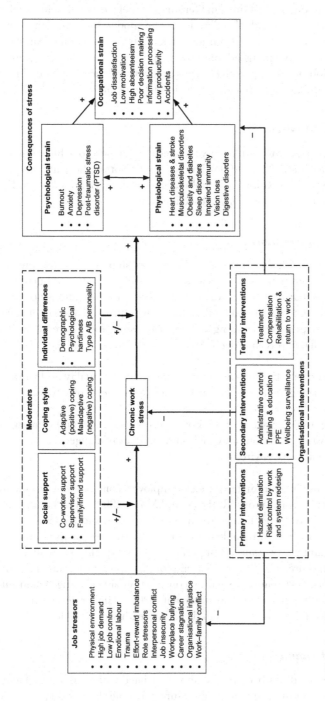

Figure 2.1 Model of work stress

stressors and strains, which are referred to as moderators. Three such moderator groups are commonly identified in literature, namely: occupational social support, copying style and individual differences. The moderators can either amplify or weaken the stress perceived from job stressors by an individual. Similarly, stress management interventions adopted by organisations can alter the presence and severity of job stressors, perceived stress and consequences suffered. The ensuing sections discuss each component of the model in detail.

Stressors at work

Stressors are physical and/or psychological demands to which an individual responds (Landy and Conte 2006). Numerous stressors in the workplace setting are identified in the occupational psychology literature, which are shown in Figure 2.1 and expounded in the following subsections.

Physical environment

Shea, Pettit and Cieri (2011) claimed a relationship between the physical work environment and such psychological issues as stress, anxiety and burnout suffered by employees, but depression was not found to have a relationship. Features of the physical work environment that have an impact on the mental health of employees include the following (Evans, Johansson and Carrere 1994; McCoy 2002; Sunindijo and Kamardeen 2017):

- ambient properties such as noise, temperature, air quality and vibration
- spatial arrangement, for instance, office layout, level of enclosure and proximity to offices
- lighting or the presence of windows (access to daylight and window views)
- unsafe work conditions and environments (fear of danger)
- unhygienic work environment.

Noise can originate from telephones, employee conversations, tools used and equipment/plant operations (Raffaello and Maass 2002). Applebaum et al. (2010) claimed a positive correlation between noise and stress, and Wickens and Hollands (2000) stated that uncontrollable noise is particularly stressful and leads to reduced motivation and performance. Temperature and air quality, particularly chemical and dust exposure, are concerns for employees exposed to weather conditions in outdoor work environments such as construction sites (Leung, Chan and Yuen 2010; Suteeraroj and Ussahawanitchakit 2008). Higher levels of stress were associated with decreased access to daylight (Leather et al. 1998).

High job demand

High job demand has been persistently associated with work stress, fatigue, anxiety and burnout in occupational literature across all the industry or professional groups around the globe (Safe Work Australia n.d.; HSE 2019). High job demand is characterised by factors such as: long, unsocial and/or unpredictable work hours, work overload, time pressure/unrealistic deadlines, pace of work, too difficult or complex tasks, lack of breaks, monotonous, unpleasant or aversive tasks, and badly designed shift systems (Michie 2002; Leka, Griffiths and Cox 2003).

Low job control

Job control refers to the level of decision latitude at one's own work; the extent that employees can exercise control on what, how, where and when they perform the tasks of their job (Glozier 2017; Landy and Conte 2006). Harvey et al. (2017) warned that jobs with high demands (increased workload and time pressure) and low control pose the greatest risk for work stress and related mental and physical illnesses. The freedom and the ability to influence matters at work that are relevant to his/her job, decide what one wants to do at work to achieve his/her goals and having adequate autonomy to carry out the job tasks without having to refer matters upwards excessively are essential parts of job control. Leung, Chan and Cooper (2015) surmised that lack of such job autonomy is directly related to work stress, decreased job satisfaction, low self-esteem and depression. Employment arrangements such as flexible time schedules and homeworking enhance the perceptions of control over one's job by helping employees balance their family and work commitments. However, homeworking may not be practicable in all industry sectors and in all professional groups; for example, a construction supervisor's presence on site is constantly required and regular homeworking may not be applicable.

Emotional labour

Emotional labour is the regulation and management of one's emotions in the workplace to meet job or organisational demands so that employees display only certain, usually pleasant, expressions during interpersonal transactions, particularly with clients/customers, regardless of what they actually feel (Jeung, Kim and Chang 2018; Landy and Conte 2006). This involves suppressing one's actual emotions and faking/showing false emotions and expressions, which require cognitive and psychological efforts and is stressful, exhausting and psychologically distressing to sustain over a long period (Landy and Conte 2006; Pugliesi and Shook 1997). Research studies have discovered consistent associations between emotional labour and a variety of adverse behaviour, psychological and health outcomes, such as loss of memory, job dissatisfaction, depersonalisation, job stress, hypertension, heart disease, emotional exhaustion, burnout and turnover intentions (Brotheridge and Grandey 2002; Zapf 2002). Emotional labour has also been shown to exacerbate cancer (Mann 2004).

Trauma

Exposure to traumatic events at work increases the risk of mental health problems such as post-traumatic stress disorder (PTSD) and depression. Occupations with regular exposure to traumatic events – such as paramedics, medical staff, police officers, fire fighters, military personnel and journalists – have a higher likelihood of this risk. For instance, a study done by Black Dog Institute revealed that 10% of emergency service personnel currently suffer from PTSD in Australia (Black Dog Institute 2018). Construction being one of the dangerous industries with higher injury and fatality rates around the world, construction personnel who sustain or witness unexpected traumatic incidents such as amputation, crushing or the death of a co-worker may develop PTSD and depression.

Effort-reward imbalance (ERI)

ERI, a composite construct of excessive effort and insufficient reward, occurs when one perceives that the reward received is insufficient for the effort invested at work (Glozier 2017). The reward can be of three forms: financial, esteem and career development (Leung, Chan and Cooper 2015). Harvey et al. (2017) claimed that the most stressful work condition is one in which ERI is persistent and an increased ERI is a greater risk factor for developing depression and anxiety disorders (Niedhammer et al. 2006; de Jonge et al. 2000).

Role stressors

Role ambiguity, role conflict and role overload are collectively referred to as role stressors (Landy and Conte 2006, p423). Role ambiguity occurs when an employee lacks clear knowledge about his/her job's responsibilities and objectives, and role conflict arises when there are conflicting expectations from an employee's role whilst role overload happens when an employee is expected to fulfil too many roles simultaneously (Harvey et al. 2017; Landy and Conte 2006). Schmidt et al. (2014) argued that role ambiguity and role conflict are linked to increased depression symptoms. Role overload can cause employees to constantly experience work overload, long work hours, lack of breaks and time pressure, leading to stress and subsequent strains such as tension, burnout, anxiety and propensity to leave the organisation (Landy and Conte 2006; Michie 2002; Day and Livingstone 2001).

Interpersonal conflict

Negative interactions with co-workers, supervisors or clients, which can range from heated arguments to subtle incidents of unfriendly behaviour, are referred to as interpersonal conflict at work (Jex 1998). These can occur for a variety of reasons, such as access to resources, perceived unfair treatment, different working styles, different opinions or attitudes, disagreements, and poor communications and misunderstandings. Interpersonal conflict is a significant work stressor, and has been linked to multiple negative employee outcomes such as: higher levels of somatic symptoms and turnover intentions (Frone 2000); frustration, anxiety and depression (Spector and Jex 1998); and job dissatisfaction and burnout (Demsky 2012).

Workplace bullying

Workplace bullying is repeated, unreasonable behaviour directed at an employee or a group of employees by another employee(s), manager or the employer (Safe Work Australia 2016). It can be specific task- or role-related or interpersonal-related. Examples of workplace bullying are (Safe Work Australia 2016):

- using abusive, insulting or offensive language or comments
- displaying aggressive and intimidating conduct
- making belittling or humiliating comments
- victimisation
- making practical jokes or initiation
- making unjustified criticism or complaints
- deliberate exclusion from work-related events
- withholding vital information that affects work performance
- setting unreasonable timelines or constantly changing deadlines
- allocating tasks that are unreasonably below or above one's skill level
- denying access to information, supervision, consultation or resources to the detriment of the employee
- spreading misinformation or malicious rumour
- changing work arrangements to deliberately inconvenience a particular employee or group
- sexual harassment.

Bullying is a strong psychological hazard and its impact is significantly strong on employees. Verkuil, Atasayi and Molendijk (2015) reported large correlations between burnout or PTSD and bullying. Similarly, Theorell et al. (2015) observed an association between workplace bullying and increased depressive symptoms.

Job insecurity

Perceived job insecurity is stressful and increases the risk of mental illness by about 30% (Glozier 2017), particularly depression (Theorell et al. 2015). A perception of job insecurity can be provoked by external economic factors or organisational change such as downsizing, restructuring, relocation, mergers, and technology and management changes (Harvey et al. 2017). Moreover, certain industry norms also raise perceptions of job insecurity. For example, in the construction industry, masculinity and male dominated roles are commonplace. Bowen, Govender and Edwards (2014) reported that women who work in this field felt job insecurity and anxiety because they needed to function compatibly to the masculine workplace and prove themselves.

Career stagnation

Prospect of career progression provides a buffer against stress experienced at work and motivates individuals to overcome challenges at work. However, under promotion as well as lack of opportunities for continual skill development and career progression can be frustrating, stressful and yield job dissatisfaction and propensity to leave. In the construction sector, women reported to have experienced challenges with career progression as a stressor because of the industry's dominant male career model (Dainty and Lingard 2006). Moreover, Arditi, Gluch and Holmdahl (2013) confirmed that career-progression-related discrimination occurs to women and ethnic minorities in the construction industry. However, in a study conducted by Sunindijo and Kamardeen (2017) both male and female rated almost equally the lack of career progression as a risk factor for their mental health.

Organisational injustice

Organisational justice refers to the fairness of rules and social norms within organisations. Three types of organisational justice are suggested in the literature, which are:

- distributive justice – concerns perceived fairness of the allocation of resources and rewards to employees within the organisation
- procedural justice – about the fairness in the process by which resources and rewards are distributed to employees within the organisation
- interactional justice – the sensitivity around the treatment of employees.

The interactional justice is subdivided into interpersonal/relational justice and informational justice. Interpersonal justice deals with the extent to which employees are treated with respect, politeness and dignity at work. Informational justice addresses the presence or absence of adequate information and communications from management about workplace procedures.

Ndjaboué, Brisson and Vézina (2012), and Nieuwenhuijsen, Bruinvels and Frings-Dresen (2010) found that low relational justice and low procedural justice were associated with increased likelihood of work stress induced mental health problems among employees, independently of other stressors such as high job demand, low job control and ERI. In the construction sector, organisational injustice centred around the age and gender has been found to cause job dissatisfaction, work stress, burnout, sleep problems and female employee turnover (Nwaogu et al. 2019; Sunindijo and Kamardeen 2017; Kamardeen and Sunindijo 2017; Bowen, Govender and Edwards 2014).

Work–life conflict

Family and work are two important elements that enable one to enjoy a good quality of life. However, when one experiences conflicts between the responsibilities of work and family, it then transpires as a stressor. Moreover, there is a bi-directional relationship between family and work; work responsibilities can affect the family life and family responsibilities can affect work (Levy 2010).

Having a good, relaxing quality of life outside work, characterised by a supportive and happy home environment and engagements in regular social and leisure activities, helps to recover from daily stress of work. However, in present days, high job demands increasingly spill out into homes and social lives of employees, affecting the recovery refuge. Long or uncertain work hours, working away from home, taking work home (often caused by deadlines and increased responsibilities/workload) and frequent travels for work may adversely affect the fulfilment of family responsibilities, available family time and engagement in social and leisure activities (Michie 2002).

Since dual-career families have become the norm rather than the exception in present societies, work–family conflict has become a pervasive stressor for both men and women. It is particularly stressful for working women because they still continue to carry more of the responsibilities within the home (Landy and Conte 2006). In a study of men and women working in high ranking positions, Lundberg and Frankenhaeuser (1999) discovered that women were more stressed due to their simultaneous family and household duties. In many instances, women may opt to work in lower paid, lower status and part-time/shift work to accommodate family responsibilities (Michie 2002). This also may turn into a stressor owing to the feelings of under-utilisation of skills and under achievements of aspirations, resulting in higher levels of stress for women.

Consequences of stress

Reactions or responses to stressors are classified into three types of strains in literature, namely: psychological, physiological and occupational.

Psychological strains

Safe Work Australia (2006) identified four common types of work-stress-related mental disorders such as: burnout, anxiety disorder, depression and PTSD.

Burnout

Burnout is a state of emotional, mental and physical exhaustion caused by excessive and prolonged stress (Jeung, Kim and Chang 2018). It is characterised by three dimensions (WHO 2019):

- feeling of exhaustion or energy depletion
- increased mental distance from one's job or negativity/cynicism towards one's job
- diminished professional efficacy.

Rossi, Quick and Perrewe (2009) postulated that a structural relationship among these dimensions that prolonged work stress causes exhaustion, leading to cynicism and diminished professional efficacy. In the context of construction professionals, long work hours are strongly associated with burnout symptoms (Lingard and Francis 2009).

Anxiety disorder

Feeling anxious is a natural reaction of the mind and body when one is confronted with a stressful situation and it ceases with the fading of the stressor. It is a normal part of life. However, anxiety disorders refer to a psychiatric condition that is characterised by intense, excessive and persistent fear or worry about a situation that poses little or no danger and interferes with daily functioning (ADAA 2018). Common symptoms include (Mayo Clinic 2018): nervousness, restlessness or irritability; having a sense of impending danger or doom; heart racing; rapid breathing; sweating; trembling; difficulty controlling worry; disturbed sleep; gastrointestinal problems; concentration difficulties; and trouble thinking of anything other than the present worry.

Akin to normal life, at work employees feel anxious occasionally when they face stressful circumstances such as deadlines, performance reviews and dealing with client complaints. However, persistent anxiety/anxiety disorders can be experienced due to the presence of certain stressors such as job insecurity, excessive workload, dangerous work and lack of control (Braverman 1992).

Depression

Depression is a psychiatric condition in which a person persistently feels lowered mood, sad, discouraged, hopeless, unmotivated or disinterested in life in general for longer than 2 weeks and the emotions interfere with daily activities. Depressive feelings are experienced by almost all from time to time when confronted with unpleasant or unhappy situations, but they disappear within days. In the case of people with depressive disorders, the feelings are intense and last for long periods, maybe weeks, months or years. Symptoms of depression appear in four dimensions as described here (Beyond Blue 2020):

- behaviour – withdrawing from close family and friends, lost interest in usual enjoyable activities, not getting things done at work, unable to concentrate, and relying on alcohol and sedatives
- feelings – overwhelmed, irritable, frustrated, unhappy, guilty, lacking confidence, indecisive and miserable
- thoughts – I'm a failure, I'm worthless, it's my fault, nothing good happens ever, life is not worth living, and people would be better off without me
- physical – fatigue, headache and muscle pains, sleep problems, loss/change of appetite, and significant weight loss or gain.

Bowen et al. (2018) maintained that high job pressure, low job autonomy and control, and work–life conflict are significant predictors of depression-related symptoms among construction professionals.

Post-traumatic stress disorder (PTSD)

PTSD can develop following an exposure to a traumatic event that threatened one's life or safety or that of others around them and they felt intense fear, horror and helplessness. Among the examples of such traumatic events are accidents, natural disasters, war, terrorism and physical or sexual assault. People with PTSD display four types of symptoms (Beyond Blue 2020):

- re-living the traumatic event – unwanted recurring memories of the event, nightmares and reactions such as sweating, palpitation or panic when reminded of the event
- overly alert or wound up – sleeping difficulties, lack of concentration, irritability and easily startled
- deliberate avoidance of activities, places, people or conversations associated with the traumatic event
- emotional numbness – loss of interest in day-to-day activities, detachment from friends and family, and diminished affection.

In the context of construction, involvement in a serious workplace accident or witnessing a death or amputation can normally cause trauma to the victims or witnesses. The traumatic feeling normally wears off within a month, but persistent feelings beyond that period may constitute PTSD.

Physiological strains

Epidemiological literature suggests many serious and chronic diseases as physiological strains of work stress. Among them are: heart diseases (Sara et al. 2018), musculoskeletal disorders (Roquelaure 2018), digestive system disorders (Howard, Giblin and Medina 2018), obesity and type 2 diabetes (Tomiyama 2019), immune system weakening (Salvagioni et al., 2017), sleep disorders (Paunio et al. 2015) and vision loss (Sabel et al. 2018). There are interplays between the psychological and the physiological strains that one reinforces the other.

Occupational strains

The combined forces of physiological and psychological strains adversely affect job performance in multiple ways, such as: job dissatisfaction, increased absenteeism, presenteeism, poor decision making/information processing, low productivity, errors and rework, increased accident and injury rates, reduced organisational commitment and motivation, diminished client/customer relationships and high employee turnover (Ajayi 2018; Salvagioni et al. 2017; Keegel, Ostry and LaMontagne 2009). For instance, in a population-based study, VicHealth (2012) discovered that 40% of employee turnover and 60% of absenteeism were caused by work stress.

Moderators of work stress

The cognitive appraisal of stress and its consequences are influenced by various factors related to individuals, which are generally referred to as moderators. The model shown in Figure 2.1 identifies three types of stress moderators and the following sections detail them.

Social support

A growing body of literature has emphasised the role of social support in reducing work stress and improving wellbeing. Social support is defined as the availability of helping relationships and the quality of those relationships (Leavy 1983, p5). At work it refers to the availability of co-workers and supervisors for support to attenuate job strain (Blanch 2016). Mueller (1980) classified social support into four types:

- affective support (also known as esteem support or emotional support) – receiving care and acceptance
- informational support – receiving guidance or advice
- instrumental support (also known as tangible aid) – receiving material assistance for specific needs
- social companionship – having people to do things with.

Research has found that social support has three types of intervening effects in the stressor–strain relationship: direct, moderator and mediator effect (Viswesvaran, Sanchez and Fisher 1999). Wang (2018) explained the mechanisms of these varying effects that social support: (1) reduces the strain experienced; (2) mitigates the perceived stressors; and (3) moderates the stressor–strain relationship.

Ross et al. (1989) suggested that social support can be drawn from four sources: supervisor, co-worker, spouse and friends/relatives. Ducharme and Martin (2000) observed that social support received from co-workers significantly contributes to job satisfaction, productivity and wellbeing, and Lingard and Francis (2006) found that social support received from co-workers and supervisors helped with the prevention of burnout due to work–life conflict. For instance, employees can cover one another in pressing situations and supervisors can provide flexibility or time off to deal with the issue (instrumental support). Moreover, receiving advice or guidance (informational support) from co-workers and/or supervisors to solve work problems is another strong social support that mitigates the negative effects of stressors. Social support from a spouse, family and friends refers to having emotionally comforting or boosting conversations, and assistance with childcare and/or household chores (instrumental support). This is particularly essential for dual-career couples (Goldsmith 2007). Wang (2018) summarised that social support alleviates burnout when it is received from different sources and in all four forms.

Coping style

Coping refers to an individual's ongoing conscious attempts to minimise or manage stressors and their negative effects (i.e. strains). Coping strategies adopted by an individual are classified into two broad categories, namely adaptive (positive) and maladaptive (negative). Positive coping strategies help diminish the stress being experienced and allow one to overcome the stressors and their negative effects successfully. Examples of adaptive strategies include (Leung, Chan and Cooper 2015; Foster 2014; Levy 2010; Carver, Scheier and Weintraub 1989):

- planful problem-solving – planning and taking active steps to remove or evade the stressor or to curtail its effects
- positive reappraisal – it is an internal cognitive adjustment process by which one restructures and reconstrues a problem positively and looks for the 'silver lining', making the best of a bad situation and tries to grow as a person
- seeking support – seeking advice, assistance or information from colleagues, people with more experience, friends or a counsellor to solve the problem or for moral support
- practising relaxation techniques – engaging in meditation, breathing exercises, sitting in/walking through nature or progressive muscle relaxation
- physical activities – engaging in team sports, exercise, yoga or swimming
- engaging in humour, fun and leisure activities such as gardening, going to the movies and socialising
- eating well-balanced meals
- resting and sleeping enough.

Negative coping strategies might help abate stress temporarily and provide a quick fix and short-term relief, but they serve to maintain mental and physiological disorders. Among the examples of maladaptive coping strategies are (Leung, Chan and Cooper 2015; Foster 2014; Levy 2010; Carver, Scheier and Weintraub 1989):

- escapism – disassociating from others and making oneself busy with work, TV, reading, internet, etc.
- numbing – consuming alcohol or drugs to forget the stressful situation
- smoking to get a temporary relief from stress
- emotional eating and drinking – consuming comfort food and drinks to get temporary relief from stress
- criticising or blaming others for the situation

- compulsive spending – frequent shopping and buying gifts for oneself to feel happy and forget stress
- denial/distancing – ignoring as if nothing happened or trying to forget the negative thing
- releasing tension by crying, yelling, throwing things, etc.

Individual differences

Clarke and Cooper (2004) argued that individuals differ in their reaction to stress and therefore individual differences play a significant role in the effects of job stress. Jick and Mitz (1985) proposed a framework of individual differences and stress processes, which was further evolved by Kamardeen and Sunindijo (2017), as depicted in Figure 2.2. The framework argues that individual differences moderate all facets of the stress process such as stress appraisal, stress coping and stress effects (strains). The moderating individual differences include demographic, psychological hardiness, self-esteem and personality type. The mechanisms as to how these factors moderate the stress process are detailed in the following sections.

Demographic

Kamardeen and Sunindijo (2017) summarised five demographic factors of employees that are likely to influence the stress process, which are: gender, age, marital status, occupation type and income level.

Women are generally highly represented in statistics related to work stress symptoms and mental disorders. For instance, Collins (2008) reported that women were more likely to file stress-related workers' compensation claims and suffer depression than men. Similarly, Kessler et al. (2005) found in epidemiological studies that women develop anxiety disorders double the rate of men. Felmingham et al. (2012) claimed that the reason for this increased representation of women is the difference in biological mechanisms between men and women. On the other hand, some other studies show that men are more vulnerable because mental

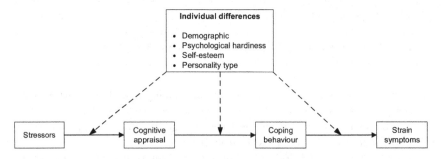

Figure 2.2 Stress and individual differences
Source: Modified from Kamardeen and Sunindijo 2017

illness is a sign of weakness and therefore hesitate to seek support whereas women are more willing to seek support (Kamardeen and Sunindijo 2017).

Although physical health depletes with age, older employees are better able to manage stressors at work due to their extended experience in the same field and therefore generally have better mental health than younger employees (Skogstad et al. 2013; Chang et al. 2006).

Married individuals reported to have generally better mental health (Amato 2015) and singles, particularly those who are separated, divorced or widowed, were found to have more symptoms of psychological distress, psychiatric disorders and psychosomatic symptoms (Thoits 2010). Amato (2015) argued that a functioning married life provides several benefits to individuals which help to restrain the adverse effects of work stress. For instance, it provides social support and extends the social networks which can be drawn upon for support or socialisation. Married individuals often have regular leisure and social activities as well as other things in life to take their mind off work stressors. Moreover, marriage increases self-esteem and social status, which helps with better coping.

Certain occupations can be more stressful than others due to their inherent nature and therefore can influence the development of stress and strain symptoms. For example, Leung, Chan and Cooper (2015) found in the construction industry of Hong Kong that construction workers and quantity surveyors showed more symptoms of stress than project managers, architects and engineers. Moreover, Thoits (2010) observed more mental health problems among those who were in occupations that are considered less prestigious.

Individuals with a low income appeared to show higher rates of psychological distress and mental disorders than those who were in a better socio-economic condition (Thoits 2010). Individuals with low incomes are likely to be enduring stressful life circumstances, accompanied by a sense of reduced control over life due to financial insecurity, and any further work stressors are likely to worsen the strain symptoms.

Psychological hardiness

Hardiness is a personality that provides stamina to withstand stress (Weinberg and Gould 2011), and to actively engage in adaptive coping strategies (Quick et al. 2013). Landy and Conte (2006) described that hardy individuals possess three characteristics:

- they feel they are in control of their lives (having an internal locus of control)
- they have a sense of commitment to their family, work goals and values
- they perceive unexpected change as a challenge rather than an obstacle.

Hardiness moderates the relationship between stressors and strains, so much so that hardy individuals reported to have fewer physiological reactions to stressors and higher levels of general wellbeing compared to less hardy people (Kobasa, Maddi and Kahn 1982).

Self-esteem

Self-esteem is an overall evaluation of one's personal worth or value. It is a collection of an individual's attitudes towards him/herself, i.e. the sum of self-confidence (a feeling of personal capacity), and self-respect (a feeling of personal worth) (Kanayo 2016). Self-esteem is a moderator of the stress–strain relationship (Cooper, Dewe and O'Driscoll 2001) as individuals with low self-esteem are likely to experience more strains and individuals with high self-esteem are more likely to adopt adaptive coping methods (Landy and Conte 2006). However, a vicious cycle is also possible between self-esteem and work stress. Self-esteem can impact one's performance and stress coping to a large extent and employees' self-esteem is negatively influenced by their failure to meet goals, and thereby work stress (Akgunduz 2013).

Personality type

Robbins et al. (2015) claimed that individual behavioural patterns affect how a person reacts to stressors and they have been found to be strong moderators in the stress–strain relationship. Friedman and Rosenman (1959) theorised two behaviour patterns, namely: type A and type B, and Table 2.1 depicts the differences in the two behaviour patterns. Type A behaviour pattern is characterised by achievement striving, time urgency and extraordinary mental and physical alertness, and type B is the complete opposite, with characteristics of the absence of drive, ambition and sense of urgency (Kamardeen and Sunindijo 2017).

Hallberg, Johansson and Schaufeli (2007) postulated that individuals who demonstrated high type A behaviour patterns were excellent performers but

Table 2.1 Individual behaviour patterns (modified from Clarke and Cooper 2004)

Type A behaviour pattern	*Type B behaviour pattern*
• Always on time	• Casual about time keeping
• Very competitive	• Not competitive
• Anticipates what others are going to say, nods and attempts to finish	• Good listener
• Always rushed	• Never feels rushed, even when under pressure
• Impatient while waiting	• Can wait patiently
• Tries to do many things at once, thinks about what will do next	• Takes things one at a time
• Emphatic in speech, fast and forceful	• Slow, deliberate talker
• Wants a good job recognised by others	• Cares about satisfying oneself, no matter what
• Fast eating, walking, etc.	• Slow doing things
• Hard driving, pushing oneself and others	• Easy-going
• Hide feelings	• Express feelings
• Few interests outside home/work	• Many outside interests
• Ambitious	• Unambitious
• Eager to get things done	• Casual about deadlines

there was a strong relationship between this behaviour pattern and work stress. Similarly, Jamal (1999) observed that those with type A personality were more severely affected by the negative consequences of high job stress such as burnout and turnover intention. Moreover, Friedman and Rosenman (1974) noted frequent links between type A personality and coronary heart disease and heart attack, a physiological outcome of chronic stress.

Organisational stress intervention

The preceding section described how the perception of stress and its consequences are moderated by individual employees and interventions deployed by them. This section explores how organisations should intervene the stressor, stress and strain pathway to control negative effects on employees and on the organisation in general.

Safe Work Australia (2019) argued that preventing and controlling work stress is a proactive, systematic process that needs to follow four steps, as in any risk management cycle, which are:

- identifying psychosocial hazards (workplace stressors)
- assessing risk
- controlling risk
- reviewing hazards and revising control measures.

The identification of psychosocial hazards may be achieved by the following mechanisms in an organisation:

- conversations with employees, supervisors, managers and workplace wellbeing specialists
- workplace inspections/audits to observe the implementation of work activities and employee interactions
- surveying employees, supervisors and managers
- reviewing incident reports, workers' compensation claims and staff turnover reports.

Once the psychosocial hazards have been identified, the risk assessment exercise should evaluate the frequency and intensity of exposure to each identified psychosocial hazard and determine:

- the severity of risk to the wellbeing of employees exposed and the level of urgency required to address the stressor
- suitable control measures.

Controlling psychosocial hazards in the workplace should follow the same system of hierarchy of control as applied in physical hazard control, which identifies the following hierarchical order of implementation:

- eliminating psychosocial hazards
- minimising risk by applying substitution, isolation or engineering controls in work and workplace design
- administrative control of psychosocial hazard through workplace behaviour policies, and procedures and training on stress management
- personal protective equipment – examples are providing personal distress alarms, equipment to prevent stress caused by environmental factors such as noise or heat.

VicHealth (2012) proposed a three-tier model of workplace interventions for managing work stress in organisations and the tiers are named primary, secondary and tertiary level interventions. The model embodies the hierarchy of risk control discussed earlier in the first two tiers while introducing reactive measures on the third tier of intervention. Table 2.2 presents an extended version of the VicHealth model.

The last stage in the organisational stress management cycle is the review of hazards and control measures. The review can occur when: (1) a new hazard or risk emerges, (2) a control measure does not minimise the risk, (3) changes occur in the work environment and system, (4) consultation with employees suggests a review is required, or (5) a wellbeing representative requests a review.

Research method

The preceding sections explained the causes, consequences, moderators and interventions of work stress from a general occupational psychology perspective. However, not every stressor is relevant to every industrial sector and the manifestation of these stressors can vary across industries depending on the nature of the business. In the context of construction, some listed stressors may be more relevant and strongly present than others. Moreover, the nature of organisational interventions can vary depending on whether it is a site-based or office-based work environment. Hence, the remainder of this chapter investigates the Australian construction industry context in detail and tests the applicability of the work stress model presented in Figure 2.1. Accordingly, the following research questions are investigated empirically:

- What is the degree of prevalence of work stress induced psychological disorders among construction professionals, and due to different socio-demographic characteristics of construction professionals?
- What are the significant job stressors that predict the poor psychological conditions? What stress coping methods do construction professionals adopt, and how do these influence psychological health outcomes?
- What interventions do organisations in the construction industry apply to control work stress among employees, and how do these affect mental health and job outcomes of their employees?

Table 2.2 Organisational stress management framework (modified from VicHealth 2012 and Safe Work Australia 2019)

Intervention level	Risk controls method applies	Examples of intervention objectives and actions	
		Objective	*Action*
Most effective	**Primary** Goal: to eliminate or reduce risk factors for job stress	Control at the source of psychosocial hazard or interception of the hazard in its path from source to employee through: • hazard elimination • substitution with safer approach • process isolation to contain exposure • engineering control to reduce exposure.	• Reduce job demand • Improve job control • Improve job resources • Improve social support	• Setting achievable workloads and performance targets for employees • Improving the physical work environment with appropriate equipment/technology to reduce exposure to stressors such as noise, heat and physical demand • Redesigning work and work system to: allocate adequate time and resources to complete tasks, particularly for difficult tasks performed by less-experienced employees • match work allocation with appropriate staff • minimise confusion in employees' roles, reporting structures and performance standards • provide employees with control over their work pace, schedule and preferences • increase practical support during peak workload • increase employee participation in work planning and decision making • Integrate individual employee needs to optimise supervisory social support • Create clear promotion pathways.

(*continued*)

Table 2.2 Cont.

Intervention level	Risk controls method applies	Examples of intervention objectives and actions	
		Objective	Action
Secondary Goal: to alter the ways individuals perceive or respond to stressors	Control at the individual employee level through: • administrative controls • training and education • personal protective equipment • wellbeing surveillance.	• Alter individual responses to job stressors • Improve individual ability to cope with short-term stress responses • Detect stress-related symptoms and intervene early	• Provide right information, training and supervision to employees to do their job well • Provide cognitive behavioural therapy or relaxation response training to employees • Provide anger management training • Conduct health screening for stress symptoms, ambulatory blood pressure and hypertension • Ensure workplace values and reward systems that support collaboration, teamwork and peer support • Train supervisors on people and work management, on the job support and to recognise early warning symptoms of psychological injury/first aid in mental health
Least effective **Tertiary** Goal: to treat, compensate and rehabilitate employees with job-stress-related illness	Control at the level of illness through: • treatment • workers' compensation • rehabilitation and return to work programs.	• Treat job-stress-related illness • Compensate job-stress-related illness • Rehabilitate job stress affected employees	• Provide medical care, counselling and employee assistance programs • Reduce adversarial aspects of compensation process • Include modification of job stressors in return-to-work plans

Data

The dataset required for this research was extracted from the complete data collected from the Australian construction industry using an online questionnaire survey. The details of the survey, its administration and respondents were discussed in Chapter 1, under the 'research methodology' section, and therefore are not repeated in this chapter, but the data pertinent to this chapter are summarised in Table 2.3. Moreover, a copy of the complete survey instrument can be found in the Appendix.

There were 310 participants who responded to the survey, but only 247 responses were complete and could be used for analysis. This was above the minimum required sample size of 241 for a survey that collects responses on a 4-point Likert scale, as per Park and Jung (2009). Refer to Table 1.3 in Chapter 1 for socio-demographic details of the survey respondents. Except for the socio-demographic details of the respondents, responses to most other questions were collected on 4-point textual Likert scales. The textual Likert scales used in the survey were coded numerically in the following manner to standardise and facilitate quantitative analyses:

- Scale 1: never = 0, sometimes = 1, often = 2, always = 3
- Scale 2: not satisfied = 0, somewhat satisfied = 1, satisfied = 2, very satisfied = 3
- Scale 3: never = 0, once or twice = 1, monthly = 2, weekly = 3
- Scale 4: not at all = 0, several days = 1, more than half the days = 2, nearly every day = 3

Moreover, constructs such as work–life conflict and job stress were measured by multiple items in the questionnaire. In order to ensure that the measurement items adequately represent the constructs, internal consistency and reliability tests were conducted with Cronbach's alpha tests. Moreover, statistical means for the constructs were computed for use in further analyses. Table 2.4 depicts the results. To accept that a construct is reliable and the measurement items within a construct are internally consistent, the Cronbach's α value must be higher than .70 (Tavakol and Dennick 2011). The constructs yielded alpha values of greater than the threshold.

Data analysis techniques

A variety of analysis techniques were used to answer the questions on page 34:

- The prevalence of psychological disorders was assessed using descriptive statistics, along with inferential techniques such as one-sample t-tests for population. Moreover, Kruskal-Wallis H tests were performed to investigate how the differences in socio-economic factors influence psychological health outcomes.

Table 2.3 Data pertinent to work stress induced psychological disorders

Section	Response options

Respondent's background

1. Gender (male, female or other)

2. Age (≤20, 21–30, 31–40, 41–50, 51–60 or >60)

3. Marital status (married/de-facto, single or divorced/separated/widowed)

4. Organisation type (property development, PM, architecture, engineering, QS, builder, subcontractor, FM or other)

5. Organisation size (measured by # of full-time employees) (≤4, 5–19, 20–199 or ≥200)

6. Job title (text responses were received but categorised as junior professional, mid-career professional, senior professional or executive)

7. Experience (<1 year, 1–5 years, 6–10 years or >10 years)

8. Nature of employment (permanent, fixed-term contract or casual)

9. Hours worked weekly (<20, 20–30, 30–40, 40–50 or >50)

10. Workplace environment (site or office)

11. Income (<$40k, $40–60k, $60–80k, $80–100k, $100–120k, $120–150k or >$150k)

Job stressors

In the past 6 months at work how often did you experience: Measured using the scale of:

1. Poor/dangerous work environment   • Never

2. Excessive workload   • Sometimes

3. Unpredictable work hours   • Often

4. Time pressure   • Always

5. Job autonomy

6. Job appropriateness

7. Flexibility

8. Supportive feedback

9. Line manager support

10. Co-worker support

11. Harassment

12. Bullying

13. Discrimination

14. Role ambiguity

15. Adequate job resources

Table 2.3 Cont.

Section	Response options
16. Staff consultation	
17. Sufficient remuneration	
18. Reward	
19. Job security	
20. Career prospect	

Work–private life conflict

In the past 6 months how often did you experience:	Measured using the scale of:
1. Lack of energy for private life	• Never
2. Lack of time for private life	• Sometimes
3. Family complained about too much work	• Often
4. Other personal life stressors	• Always

Chronic job stress

In the past 4 weeks how often did you experience:	Measured using the scale of:
1. Poor sleep	• Never
2. Restlessness	• Sometimes
3. Irritability	• Often
4. Tensed	• Always
5. Nervousness	

Stress coping methods

In the past 4 weeks how often did you engage in the following stress coping methods:	Measured using the scale of:
	• Not at all
1. Problem-solving	• Several days
2. Positive reappraisal	• More than half the days
3. Seeking support	• Nearly every day
4. Relaxation	
5. Physical activity	
6. Leisure and humour	
7. Eating balanced diet	
8. Adequate sleep	
9. Isolation	
10. Alcohol/drug use	

(*continued*)

Table 2.3 Cont.

Section	Response options
11. Smoking	
12. Emotional eating	
13. Criticise/blame others	
14. Compulsive spending	
15. Denial/ignoring as if nothing happened	
16. Releasing tension	

Mental health effects

A) In the past 6 months how often were you bothered by/treated for: 1. Burnout 2. Anxiety 3. Depression	Measured using the scale of: • Never • Once or twice • Monthly • Weekly
B) Do you believe that your job is the primary cause? (this was asked for each mental disorder above)	Dichotomous response –Yes / No

Job outcomes

In the past 6 months how would you rate your: 1. Job satisfaction 2. Job performance	Measured using a scale of 1 (low) to 10 (high)

Organisational interventions

In the past 6 months how often did your organisation apply the following interventions to improve employee wellbeing: 1. Improving work policies and conditions 2. Changing working conditions and practices 3. Skill improvement for employees 4. Training managers on employee wellbeing 5. Stress management training for employees 6. Facilitating relaxation and exercise programs 7. Promoting peer support 8. Psychological counselling, care & therapy 9. Rehabilitation & RTW for wellbeing issues	Measured using the scale of: • Never • Sometimes • Often • Always

Table 2.4 Reliability assessment for constructs

Construct	Items	Cronbach's α	Mean
Work–life conflict	• Lack of energy for private life • Lack of time for private life • Family complain about too much work • Other personal life stressors	.826	1.275
Work stress	• Poor sleep • Restlessness • Irritability • Tensed • Nervousness	.919	1.178

- Experiences of job stressors and stress coping methods among construction professionals were evaluated using descriptive statistics. Moreover, independent sample t-tests along with Leven's tests for homogeneity were conducted to investigate the differences between male and female professionals.
- Classification and regression tree technique was used to investigate the interactions among: (1) stressors and work stress, and (2) work stress, stress coping methods and psychological disorders.
- The level of implementation of organisational stress management interventions was assessed using descriptive statistics, but Kruskal-Wallis H tests were performed to examine how it varies across different organisation sizes. Moreover, associations between stress management interventions, and mental strain and job outcomes were explored using Pearson bi-variate correlation analysis.

Construction professionals and work-related psychological disorders

This section elaborates the data analyses and findings under pertinent headings and subheadings, which in turn address the research questions set out in the research method section.

Prevalence of psychological disorders among construction professionals

Descriptive statistical analyses were performed to understand the level of prevalence of work stress, burnout, anxiety and depression and their severities among construction industry professionals who responded to the survey. In addition to utilising the aggregate mean response discussed in Table 2.4 for work stress, participants' responses to the questions shown in Table 2.5 were analysed:

Figure 2.3 illustrates work stress prevalence among construction professionals in Australia. Ninety-three percent of the respondents claimed that they endure work stress. The mean stress experience was calculated at 1.18 for the sample

Table 2.5 Questions analysed for psychological disorders

In the past 6 months how often were you bothered by / treated for:

1) Burnout   Do you believe that job stress may have caused this illness?
   • *Never*   • Yes
   • *Once or twice*   • No
   • *Monthly*
   • *Weekly*

2) Anxiety   Do you believe that job stress may have caused this illness?
   • *Never*   • Yes
   • *Once or twice*   • No
   • *Monthly*
   • *Weekly*

3) Depression   Do you believe that job stress may have caused this illness?
   • *Never*   • Yes
   • *Once or twice*   • No
   • *Monthly*
   • *Weekly*

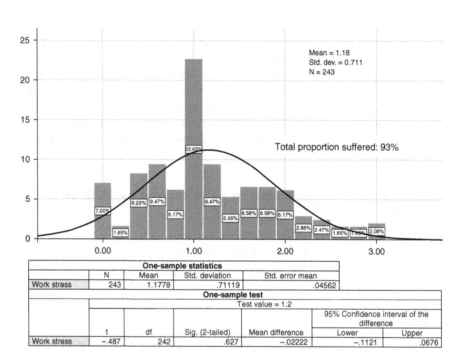

One-sample statistics				
	N	Mean	Std. deviation	Std. error mean
Work stress	243	1.1778	.71119	.04562

One-sample test						
Test value = 1.2						
					95% Confidence interval of the difference	
	t	df	Sig. (2-tailed)	Mean difference	Lower	Upper
Work stress	−.487	242	.627	−.02222	−.1121	.0676

Figure 2.3 Prevalence of work stress

surveyed. Then, one sample t-test was conducted to check whether the inferred population mean of 1.2 is significantly different from that of the sample that responded to the survey in this study. The p-value of .627, which is greater than the threshold p-value of .05, suggests that the stress level of the population of

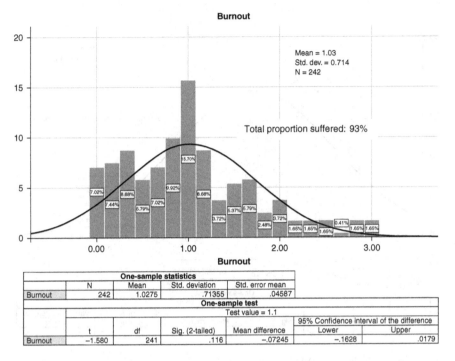

Figure 2.4 Prevalence of burnout

One-sample statistics				
	N	Mean	Std. deviation	Std. error mean
Burnout	242	1.0275	.71355	.04587

One-sample test						
			Test value = 1.1			
					95% Confidence interval of the difference	
	t	df	Sig. (2-tailed)	Mean difference	Lower	Upper
Burnout	−1.580	241	.116	−.07245	−.1628	.0179

professionals is not significantly different from that of the sample surveyed. Moreover, around one-fourth, half, and one-sixth of the industry professionals reported low, moderate and high severity levels, respectively. In total, 93% of the professionals in the construction industry suffer from work stress with varying degrees of severity.

Figure 2.4 illustrates burnout prevalence among construction professionals in Australia and 93% of the respondents claim to experience it. The mean level of burnout experienced was calculated at 1.03 for the sample surveyed. Then, one sample t-test was conducted to check whether the inferred population mean of 1.10 is significantly different from that of the sample that responded to the survey in this study. The p-value of .116, which is greater than the threshold p-value of .05, suggests that the burnout level of the population of professionals is not significantly different from that of the sample surveyed. Moreover, around 55%, 30% and 9% of the industry professionals reported low, moderate and high severity levels, respectively. In total, 93% of the professionals in the construction industry endure burnout in varying degrees. The total proportion of sufferers is the same as work stress, which demonstrates the direct close relationship between stress and burnout.

Figure 2.5 illustrates the prevalence of work induced anxiety among construction professionals in Australia. Fifty-eight percent of respondents indicated that they suffer from anxiety and they further claimed that it is work induced. The mean

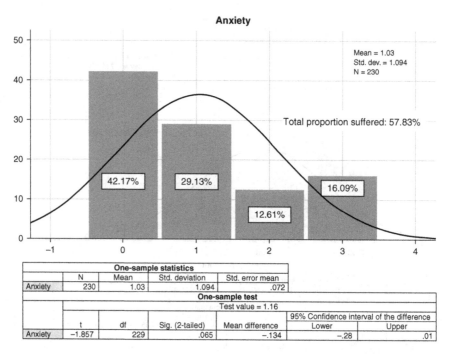

Anxiety

Mean = 1.03
Std. dev. = 1.094
N = 230

Total proportion suffered: 57.83%

42.17%   29.13%   16.09%   12.61%

One-sample statistics				
	N	Mean	Std. deviation	Std. error mean
Anxiety	230	1.03	1.094	.072

One-sample test						
Test value = 1.16						
					95% Confidence interval of the difference	
	t	df	Sig. (2-tailed)	Mean difference	Lower	Upper
Anxiety	−1.857	229	.065	−.134	−.28	.01

Figure 2.5 Prevalence of anxiety

level of anxiety experienced was calculated at 1.03 for the sample surveyed. Then, one sample t-test was conducted to check whether the inferred population mean of 1.16 is significantly different from that of the sample that responded to the survey in this study. The p-value of .065, which is greater than the threshold p-value of .05, suggests that the anxiety level of the population of professionals is not significantly different from that of the sample surveyed. Moreover, around one-third, one-eighth and one-sixth of the industry professionals reported low, moderate and high severity levels of anxiety, respectively. In total, around 58% of the professionals in the con-struction industry experience work stress induced anxiety at varying degrees.

Figure 2.6 illustrates the prevalence of depression among construction professionals in Australia. Forty-seven percent of the survey respondents claimed to experience it and it is induced by work. The mean level of depression experienced was calculated at .81 for the sample surveyed. One-sample t-test was conducted to check whether the inferred population mean of .9 is significantly different from that of the sample that responded to the survey in this study. The p-value of .185, which is greater than the threshold p-value of .05, suggests that the depression level of the population of professionals is not significantly different from that of the sample surveyed. Moreover, around one-fourth, one-eighth and one-eighth of the industry professionals reported low, moderate and high severity levels of

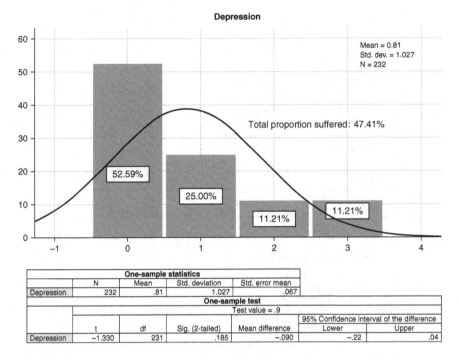

Figure 2.6 Prevalence of depression

depression, respectively. In total, almost half of the professionals in the construction industry experience depression at varying levels of severity.

Previous studies that were conducted some time ago discovered that nearly
70% of construction professionals suffer from stress, anxiety or depression (CIOB
2006). This study provides a more detailed outlook to the prevalence and updates
the figure reported previously. Ninety-three percent of construction professionals
suffer from stress and the percentage is reduced to around 60% and 50% for
anxiety and depression sufferers, respectively. Few studies on burnout among
construction professionals are notable. Leung, Chan and Dongyu (2011) found
that construction project managers in Hong Kong suffered burnout due to job
stress. Similarly, Lingard and Francis (2004) studied burnout among construction
professionals in Australia. However, these studies did not establish a percentage of
total sufferers. The present study adds a new piece of knowledge that 93% of construction professionals endure burnout. The total proportion is the same as stress
sufferers, though there is a clear difference in the spread of severity levels between
stress and burnout. It is evident that work stress and burnout are the predominant psychological strains suffered, followed by anxiety and depression among
construction professionals in Australia.

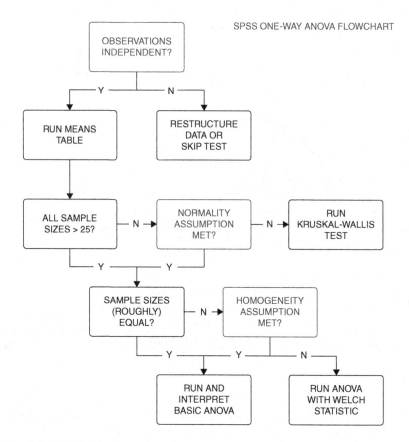

Figure 2.7 ANOVA flowchart

Source: SPSS-Tutorials.com, www.spss-tutorials.com/spss-one-way-anova/

Influence of socio-demographic factors

The influence of socio-demographic factors on psychological strain experiences were assessed using Kruskal-Wallis tests. The flowchart shown in Figure 2.7 explains the process of robustly undertaking tests for group differences. In order to run ANOVA (analysis of variance) tests, the groups need to meet criteria such as normality, minimum group size of 25 and equal group sizes. However, the groups within the respondents for different socio-demographic factors did not meet these criteria. Hence, non-parametric Kruskal-Wallis tests were undertaken. The gender, age, experience, occupation level and the organisation size of the respondents were used as fixed factors. Table 2.6 presents the test results. The p-values yielded for organisation size and occupation level are above .05 for all groups, suggesting that differences in the age, work experience, occupation level and the organisation size of the respondents do not demonstrate statistically significant differences in psychological strains reported. However, gender differences demonstrate an effect on anxiety and depression suffered though not on work stress and burnout.

The findings of this analysis contradict some previous studies. In the Australian context, Kamardeen and Sunindijo (2017) found among construction professionals that marital status was a vital moderator of work stress whereby professionals with a status of separated, divorced or widowed were at high risk of suffering severe anxiety, depression and acute stress; and female professionals at middle management levels reported mild to moderate anxiety and depression, whereas their male counterparts were largely within normal ranges. Sunindijo and Kamardeen (2017) argued that women professionals suffer more anxiety and acute stress symptoms than men professionals, but no significant difference was apparent between the genders in the level of depression suffered. On the contrary, Loosemore and Waters (2004) had reported that men professionals experienced slightly higher levels of stress than women in the Australian construction industry. In a different perspective, Love, Edwards and Irani (2010) claimed that those who work on site reported greater levels of stress than office-based consultants. In the South African construction industry, Bowen et al. (2018) posited that less experienced, female and low-ranking professionals were more vulnerable to psychological distress. In a previous study, Bowen, Edwards and Lingard (2013) found that architects, more than engineers, quantity surveyors and project and construction managers; and female, more than male, professionals felt stressed. The present study observes no statistically significant differences in work stress, burnout, anxiety and depression due to differences in age, experience, occupation level or organisation size. Only the gender difference demonstrated a statistically significant difference in anxiety and depression, i.e. female professionals suffer higher levels of anxiety and depression but there is no significant difference in the level of work stress and burnout endured.

Predictors of work stress in construction

Table 2.7 shows the workplace stressors that contribute to the previously mentioned prevalence of psychological strains among construction professionals in Australia. The statements used in the survey were aimed to capture the prevalence of stressors and were worded in positive and negative directions in connotation. Hence, higher mean values for some statements and lower mean values for other statements meant higher prevalence of stressors. In order to determine the top stressors, the midpoint of the scale, which is 1.50, was used as a reference since it represents both the negative and positive statements in the same manner. Accordingly, the distance by which the mean yielded for a negative statement exceeded the midpoint of 1.5 was considered to determine the strength of the stressor. Likewise, the distance by which the mean yielded for a positive statement fell below the midpoint of 1.5 was considered to determine the strength of the stressor. Consequently, six top stressors were identified such as excessive workload, unpredictable work hours, harassment, bullying, role ambiguity and lack of

Table 2.6 Socio-demographic factors and psychological strains

Gender difference vs psychological strain

	Gender	N	Mean rank	Null hypothesis	Kruskal-Wallis H	Sig.	Decision
Work stress	Male	189	118.44	Work stress level is the same across genders	2.648	.266	Retain null hypothesis
	Female	51	132.92				
	Other	3	160.33				
Burnout	Male	188	116.11	Burnout level is the same across genders	5.933	.051	Retain null hypothesis
	Female	51	138.06				
	Other	3	177.50				
Anxiety	Male	178	108.90	Anxiety level is the same across genders	**8.971**	**.011**	**Reject null hypothesis**
	Female	50	139.06				
	Other	2	114.00				
Depression	Male	179	111.14	Depression level is the same across genders	**6.440**	**.040**	**Reject null hypothesis**
	Female	50	133.18				
	Other	3	158.17				

Age difference vs psychological strain

	Gender	N	Mean rank	Null hypothesis	Kruskal-Wallis H	Sig.	Decision
Work stress	Below 20	1	107.00	Work stress level is the same across different age groups	3.687	.595	Retain null hypothesis
	20 to 30	74	118.53				
	31 to 40	59	134.39				
	41 to 50	58	118.55				
	51 to 60	32	121.19				
	Over 60	18	102.33				
Burnout	Below 20	1	63.50	Burnout level is the same across different age groups	10.246	.069	Retain null hypothesis
	20 to 30	74	124.06				
	31 to 40	59	135.53				
	41 to 50	57	119.55				
	51 to 60	32	115.11				
	Over 60	18	79.03				
Anxiety	Below 20	1	211.50	Anxiety level is the same across different age groups	3.516	.621	Retain null hypothesis
	20 to 30	70	119.79				
	31 to 40	56	110.76				
	41 to 50	55	116.33				
	51 to 60	30	107.60				
	Over 60	17	112.35				
Depression	Below 20	1	151.50	Depression level is the same across different age groups	3.742	.587	Retain null hypothesis
	20 to 30	70	105.41				
	31 to 40	58	116.97				
	41 to 50	55	123.69				
	51 to 60	30	123.12				
	Over 60	17	116.76				

(continued)

Table 2.6 Cont.

Gender difference vs psychological strain

Experience difference vs psychological strain

	Experience	N	Mean rank	Null hypothesis	Kruskal-Wallis H	Sig	Decision
Work stress	Less than 1 year	29	97.47	Work stress level is the same across different experience levels	3.969	.265	Retain null hypothesis
	1 to 5 years	115	124.17				
	6 to 10 years	37	126.12				
	Over 10 years	61	125.09				
Burnout	Less than 1 year	29	109.09	Burnout level is the same across different experience levels	2.329	.507	Retain null hypothesis
	1 to 5 years	114	123.59				
	6 to 10 years	37	131.82				
	Over 10 years	61	115.25				
Anxiety	Less than 1 year	27	121.72	Anxiety level is the same across different experience levels	1.547	.672	Retain null hypothesis
	1 to 5 years	108	109.99				
	6 to 10 years	36	115.21				
	Over 10 years	58	121.07				
Depression	Less than 1 year	27	118.67	Depression level is the same across different experience levels	5.549	.136	Retain null hypothesis
	1 to 5 years	110	107.39				
	6 to 10 years	36	116.78				
	Over 10 years	58	130.61				

Occupation level difference vs psychological strains

	Occupation level	N	Mean rank	Null hypothesis	Kruskal-Wallis H	Sig.	Decision
Work stress	Junior	62	118.35	Work stress level is the same across different professional levels	1.493	.684	Retain null hypothesis
	Mid-career	57	111.18				
	Senior	79	125.53				
	Executive	39	118.24				
Burnout	Junior	61	127.93	Burnout level is the same across different professional levels	2.042	.564	Retain null hypothesis
	Mid-career	57	110.44				
	Senior	79	116.62				
	Executive	39	119.33				
Anxiety	Junior	56	111.59	Anxiety level is the same across different professional levels	.172	.982	Retain null hypothesis
	Mid-career	55	111.40				
	Senior	76	112.14				
	Executive	37	116.24				
Depression	Junior	57	115.05	Depression level is the same across different professional levels	2.465	.482	Retain null hypothesis
	Mid-career	55	103.04				
	Senior	76	116.26				
	Executive	38	120.79				

(continued)

Table 2.6 Cont.

Gender difference vs psychological strain

Organisation size difference vs psychological strains

	Organisation size	N	Mean rank	Null hypothesis	Kruskal-Wallis H	Sig.	Decision
Work stress	Employees ≤4	22	123.25	Work stress level is the same across different organisation sizes	2.637	.451	Retain null hypothesis
	5 to 19	43	129.72				
	20 to199	77	127.36				
	Employees≥200	100	113.07				
Burnout	Employees ≤4	22	112.07	Burnout level is the same across different organisation sizes	7.573	.056	Retain null hypothesis
	5 to 19	43	142.13				
	20 to199	76	126.69				
	Employees≥200	100	109.56				
Anxiety	Employees ≤4	21	117.24	Anxiety level is the same across different organisation sizes	3.588	.310	Retain null hypothesis
	5 to 19	41	117.77				
	20 to199	74	124.11				
	Employees≥200	93	106.02				
Depression	Employees ≤4	21	133.93	Depression level is the same across different organisation sizes	4.008	.261	Retain null hypothesis
	5 to 19	41	111.22				
	20 to199	74	122.25				
	Employees≥200	95	109.23				

Table 2.7 Stressor prevalence

Stressor	Full sample (N = 244)		Male (N = 192)		Female (N = 52)		t-test
	Mean	S	Mean	S	Mean	S	p-value
Negatively worded stressors:							
I had to work in poor or dangerous physical work conditions	.32	.563	.34	.592	.27	.448	.457
I had excessive workload	1.46	.835	1.46	.837	1.44	.777	.901
I had unpredictable working hours	1.51	.801	1.54	.792	1.37	.768	.166
I had excessive time pressures	1.16	.832	1.22	.791	.92	.904	.021
I was subject to harassment in the form of unkind/unwanted words or behaviour at work	1.70	.888	1.68	.879	1.81	.908	.366
I was subject to bullying at work	1.60	.918	1.64	.807	1.72	.825	.500
I was subject to discrimination due to my gender, age or ethnic background	.38	.639	.34	.565	.52	.828	.136
I experienced work-life conflict	1.28	.686	1.26	.673	1.33	.722	.498
Positively worded stressors:							
I had a choice/say in deciding how I do my work	1.85	.873	1.86	.870	1.85	.872	.892
The work I performed was appropriate for my skills and abilities	2.28	.715	2.29	.693	2.23	.807	.621
I had flexibility with my working time	1.98	.800	2.05	.756	1.75	.926	.037
I was given supportive feedback on the work I do	1.66	.831	1.68	.830	1.58	.848	.420
I could rely on my line manager to help me out with a work problem	1.63	.991	1.70	.949	1.42	1.091	.069
If work got difficult, my colleagues helped me	1.78	.981	1.77	.992	1.84	.946	.641
I was clear what my duties and responsibilities were	.29	.608	.25	.541	.40	.774	.182
I had enough resources to go do my work	.31	.580	.23	.534	.54	.641	.002
I was consulted on matters/change that affected my job	1.45	.922	1.49	.910	1.29	.977	.155
My salary was sufficient for the work I had to do	1.65	.937	1.72	.940	1.42	.915	.044
I had job security	2.06	.895	2.05	.902	2.15	.849	.445
I received reward/appreciation for the efforts I put into my work	1.80	.876	1.79	.883	1.88	.784	.463
I had career progress opportunities	1.55	.975	1.56	1.003	1.54	.851	.886

resources. Work–life conflict was considered as a separate construct (see Table 2.6) and identified as a top stressor as well.

The preceding section demonstrated that gender has an influence on the psychological strain experiences. Stressors are the causes of psychological strains. Therefore, separate means for males and females were computed and then compared using two independent sample t-tests. The subsamples were significantly different in size. Hence, p-values of Levene's test for homogeneity of subsamples were assessed to accept the p-value for t-tests with equal variance assumed. When the p-values of Levene's tests were less than .05, p-values for t-tests with equal variance not assumed were accepted. The last column of Table 2.7 shows the recorded p-values of independent sample t-tests. The results show that there are no statistically significant differences in the experience of male and female professionals with many stressors, except for four, which are: time pressure, time flexibility, resource availability and salary. Male professionals feel that they are more pressured by time, have less flexibility and less resources for the job than their counterpart. Female professionals on the other hand report lesser satisfaction with their salary compared to males.

Previously, Sunindijo and Kamardeen (2017) reported that female professionals experienced the following stressors more than males: discrimination, bullying and sexual harassment. They further observed that male professionals experienced the following stressors more than their counterpart: unpredictable work hours, working night shifts, financial challenges (related to salary) and poor conditions of machinery. Olofsdotter and Randevåg (2016) claimed that adopting and adjusting to the masculine culture of the construction industry was straining for female professionals, and Dainty and Lingard (2006) asserted that women were faced with a lack of career progression in the construction industry. The present study does not find statistically significant comparisons to confirm or reject these claims. Rather, it highlights new points of differences.

The interaction of stressors and socio-demographic factors in producing work stress experiences was analysed using a decision tree. Song and Lu (2015) argued that decision trees are one of the most effective analytic techniques because they are: easy to use, non-parametric techniques that can handle skewed datasets (do not require normally distributed data) and robust even in the presence of missing values. Owing to these qualities, decision trees are widely used in many disciplines such as medicine, computer science, psychology, business and marketing (Ramaswami and Bhaskaran 2010). Decision trees are primarily developed for classification-based predictions; however, several other tasks are possible with them as follows (IBM Corporation 2012, pp1–2):

- **segmentation** – identify persons or objects that are likely to be members with a particular group
- **stratification** – assign cases into one of several categories, such as high, medium or low risk groups
- **prediction** – create rules and use them for predicting future events

- **data reduction and variable screening** – select a useful subset of predictors from a large set of variables for use in building a formal parametric model
- **interaction identification** – identify relationships that pertain to specific subgroups and specify these in a formal parametric model
- **category merging and discretising continuous variables** – recode group predictor categories and continuous variables with minimal loss of information.

Decision trees are induced by machine learning algorithms automatically from past data. Four statistical algorithms are widely utilised, namely: Classification and Regression Trees (CART/CRT), Chi-squares Automatic Interaction Detection (CHAID), C5.0, and Quick, Unbiased, Efficient Statistical Tree (QUEST). Table 2.8 compares these algorithms on five features. CRT algorithm was chosen for analysis in this chapter because the dependent variables analysed were continuous in nature and C5.0 algorithm is not available in IBM SPSS 26.

CRT was induced on the survey data by defining the stressors and the gender as independent, and work stress as dependent variables. Figure 2.8 illustrates the resulted classification and regression tree with variable interaction details and

Table 2.8 Comparison of statistical algorithms for decision tree induction

Algorithm	Features				
	Dependent variable suitable	*Independent variable suitable*	*Split type at each node*	*Measure used for splitting*	*Pruning technique used*
CRT	Categorical, continuous	Categorical, continuous	Binary	Gini index	Pre-pruning using a single pass algorithm
CHAID	Categorical	Categorical, continuous	Multiple	Chi-square	Pre-pruning using chi-square test for independence
C5.0	Categorical, continuous	Categorical, continuous	Multiple	Entropy info-gain	Pre-pruning using a single pass algorithm
QUEST	Categorical	Categorical, continuous	Binary	Chi-square for categorical variables; J-way ANOVA for continuous/ ordinal variables	Post-pruning

Source: Modified from Song and Lu 2015

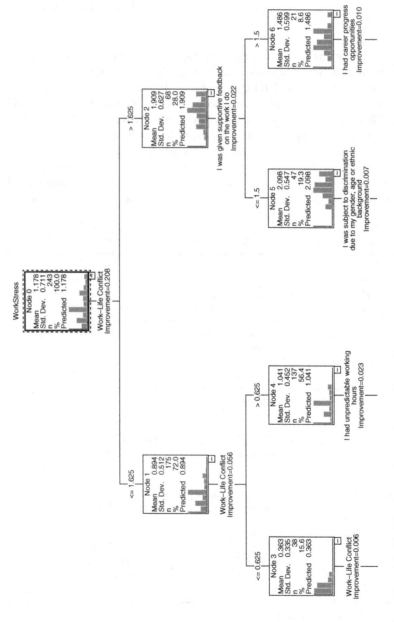

Figure 2.8 Classification and regression tree for work stress

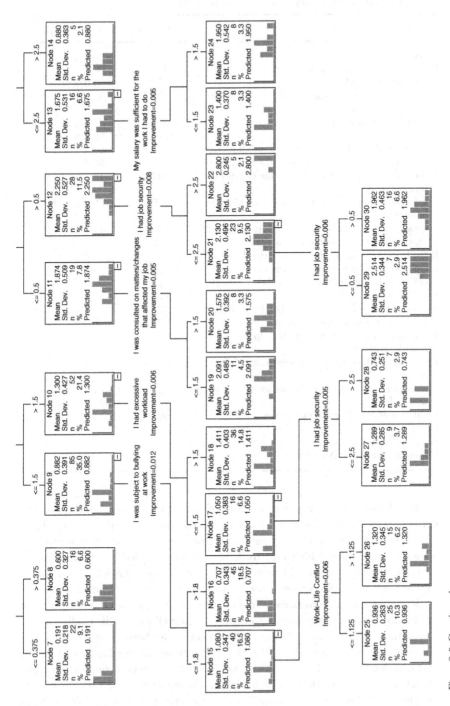

Figure 2.8 Continued

Table 2.9 Independent variable importance for work stress

Independent variable	Importance	Normalised importance
Work–life conflict	.297	100.0%
I had unpredictable working hours	.167	56.2%
I had excessive workload	.152	51.0%
I was subject to discrimination due to my gender, age or ethnic background	.093	31.2%
I was subject to bullying at work	.075	25.2%
I had job security	.067	22.5%
I was clear what my duties and responsibilities were	.064	21.4%
I was given supportive feedback on the work I do	.054	18.0%
I received reward/appreciation for the efforts I put into my work	.042	14.0%
I had to work in poor or dangerous physical work conditions	.040	13.4%
I was subject to harassment in the form of unkind/ unwanted words or behaviour at work	.033	11.2%
If work got difficult, my colleagues helped me	.030	10.0%
I had enough resources to go do my work	.028	9.6%
I had a choice/say in deciding how I do my work	.027	9.2%
I had excessive time pressures	.026	8.7%
My salary was sufficient for the work I had to do	.025	8.4%
I had career progress opportunities	.024	8.0%
I could rely on my line manager to help me out with a work problem	.023	7.7%
I was consulted on matters/changes that affected my job	.018	5.9%
The work I performed was appropriate for my skills and abilities	.013	4.3%
I had flexibility with my working time	.009	3.0%
Gender	.003	.9%

Growing Method: CRT
Dependent Variable: Work Stress

Table 2.9 identifies the key determinants of work stress. Several insights can be derived from the decision tree. Although 22 independent variables were input for predicting work stress, only nine are considered as significant determinants of work stress level, which are: work–life conflict, unpredictable work hours, excessive workload, discrimination, bullying, supportive feedback (psychological support), job insecurity, career prospect and salary. Work–life conflict appears to be the prime reason for work stress and the decision tree produced three groups of professionals based on the mean severity level yielded for work–life conflict: group 1 with mean values ≤.625, group 2 with mean values between .625 and 1.625, and group 3 with mean values ≥1.625. These can be classified as low, moderate and high levels of work–life conflict. Around 16% of construction professionals reported the lowest work stress with a mean severity level of .363 on a scale ranging from 0 to 3 who were also found to have the lowest work–life conflict severity.

For others, the combination of work–life conflict with other stressors produces varying work stress outcomes in the following manners:

- Those who have good opportunities for career progression and good supportive feedback on their work (psychological support), report low work stress despite their higher level of work–life conflict. However, only a very small proportion of professionals have these circumstances; around 2% of the population.
- Those professionals with high work–life conflict, good psychological support and high satisfaction with the salary but moderate career development opportunities in their job display high stress levels.
- Work stress level is the highest among professionals who report high work–life conflict, low job security, low supportive feedback at work and a relatively higher level of discrimination.
- Work stress level is moderate among those professionals who experience high work–life conflict and low supportive feedback but relatively lower levels of discrimination.
- The combination of moderate work–life conflict, high unpredictable work hours and excessive workload leads to moderate stress levels.
- Those with moderate work–life conflict, high unpredictable work hours and moderately excessive workload but a secure job report low work stress levels.
- Moderate work–life conflict combined with moderate unpredictable work hours and bullying produce moderate work stress levels.

Chan, Nwaogu and Naslund (2020) systematically reviewed the existing body of knowledge on mental health in the construction industry and summarised seven key risk factors for mental ill-health. These were:

- high job demand – concerns the nature of work, hours worked per week, work overload and work speed (Al-Maskari et al. 2011; Love, Edwards and Irani 2010)
- lack of job control – characterised by limited job autonomy (opportunities for decision making), office politics, authoritarian culture, strict work schedules, inconsistent communication flow and imbalanced work allocation (Lim et al. 2018; Boschman et al. 2013; Sutherland and Davidson 1993)
- work–family conflict (Sunindijo and Kamardeen 2017; Lingard et al. 2007)
- employment concerns – related to job insecurity, low income and lack of career development (Lim et al. 2018; Kamardeen and Sunindijo 2017; Bowen, Govender and Edwards 2014; Al-Maskari et al. 2011)
- workplace injustice – described by discrimination, harassment, bullying and lack of respect from subordinates (Kamardeen and Sunindijo 2017; Bowen, Govender and Edwards 2014)
- lack of support at work from colleagues and/or the line manager (Love, Edwards and Irani 2010)

- work hazards – dangerous work, and pain, injuries and illnesses associated with work (Jacobsen et al. 2013; Hu et al. 2013).

Slightly different theories exist as to which are the strongest stressors in the construction industry. Chan, Nwaogu and Naslund (2020) identified the most prominent risk factors as hours worked per week (in excess of 60 hours), work overload, low opportunity to participate in decision making, work–life conflict and lack of job autonomy. Bowen, Edwards and Lingard (2013) asserted that tight deadlines and long work hours are the key determinants. Bowen, Govender and Edwards (2014) argued that the strongest predictor of work stress was work–life imbalance, which was mediated by long work hours and perceived need to prove oneself. Cattell, Bowen and Edwards (2016) claimed that critical time constraints, volume of work and inadequate salaries were critical stressors, and work–life imbalance was particularly concerning for female professionals. Sunindijo and Kamardeen (2017) observed that the critical stressors for both genders are time pressure, excessive workload, long work hours and unpleasant work environment. They further noted that women professionals experienced more discrimination, bullying and sexual harassment.

The present study identifies the following as key determinants of work stress among construction professionals, in the descending order of influence: work–life conflict, unpredictable work hours, excessive workload, discrimination, bullying, lack of supportive feedback (psychological support), job insecurity, lack of career prospects and inadequate salaries. While there is a general agreement about key stressors, most previous studies emphasised work pressure (work hours and workload) as the most prominent risk factors but the current study highlights work–family conflict. It is almost equally stressful for both genders. However, work–life conflict and work pressure can be regarded to have bi-directional causal relationships.

Moreover, the present study finds the co-existence of risk and resilience psycho-social factors within the same workplace and demonstrates how these interact to subdue perceived work stress. It can be summarised that the perception of work stress is quite fluid among construction professionals. Though one may experience severe distress from one stressor, the comfort he/she receives from another aspect of the job serves to balance/subdue the negative effect. The strongest stress subduers are career progression opportunities, satisfactory salaries, job security and workplace consultation culture.

Stress coping and its impact on mental health among construction professionals

Table 2.10 presents the stress coping methods adopted by construction professionals in Australia. The higher the mean value yielded, the higher the adoption rate of the coping method among the construction professionals. When the total sample is observed, it appears that construction professionals apply a range of adaptive stress coping methods quite regularly. At the same time, two maladaptive

Table 2.10 Stress coping methods

Coping style	Full sample		Male		Female		T-test p-value
	Mean	S	Mean	S	Mean	S	
Problem-solving (e.g. identified the source of stress and took an action to manage it)	1.02	.966	1.00	.989	1.10	.848	.511
Keeping a positive attitude (I looked for something good in what was happening in my life and tried to grow as a person as a result of the situation)	1.45	1.040	1.37	1.026	1.76	1.011	.020
Seeking external support (e.g. talked about the stressful event with a supportive person/counsellor/friend/colleague)	1.04	.954	.90	.927	1.51	.893	.000
Relaxation (e.g. engaged in meditation, breathing exercise, sitting in nature, progressive muscle relaxation)	.69	.872	.65	.873	.88	.866	.114
Physical activity (engaged in team sports, exercise, yoga or swimming)	1.08	.985	1.05	.996	1.22	.963	.278
Engaged in humour, fun and leisure activities (gardening, movie, socialising)	1.34	.868	1.33	.878	1.39	.837	.679
Eating well-balanced meals	1.75	.954	1.72	.959	1.90	.918	.241
Resting and sleeping enough	1.34	.964	1.36	.973	1.33	.944	.851
Escape – isolating from others and making yourself busy with TV, reading, internet, etc.	1.43	1.009	1.35	1.023	1.76	.855	.012
Numbing – consuming alcohol or drugs to forget the stressful situation	.79	.951	.76	.940	.92	.954	.286
Smoking to get a relief from stress	.31	.770	.34	.782	.15	.618	.074
Emotional eating and drinking (eating comfort food and/or drinking coffee and other caffeine drinks to get relief from stress)	1.17	1.074	.99	1.031	1.79	.999	.000
Criticising or blaming others for the situation	.78	.937	.68	.895	1.15	.967	.002
Compulsive spending – shopping and buying gifts for yourself to feel happy and forget stress	.47	.667	.39	.623	.77	.751	.000
Ignoring as if nothing happened/try to forget the whole thing (denial/distancing)	.76	.915	.76	.926	.77	.905	.950
Releasing tension by crying, yelling, throwing things, etc.	.35	.666	.28	.611	.66	.788	.003

coping methods are rampant too, which are social isolation and emotional eating. Previously, Sunindijo and Kamardeen (2017) commented that both male and female construction professionals adopt problem-solving and positive reappraisal strategies quite regularly. Similarly, Love, Edwards and Irani 2010 argued that wishful thinking (positive reappraisal) and problem-solving are the predominant stress coping methods among construction professionals. The present study's findings agree with these but reveal further positive coping approaches prevalent among construction professionals. On negative coping, Roche et al. (2015) and Frone (2000) claimed that alcohol, drug and substance abuse is a common practice used for stress coping in construction. However, the present study does not find it to be rampant in the Australian construction industry.

Akin to stressors, separate means for males and females were computed and then were compared using two independent sample t-tests. The last column in Table 2.9 shows the p-values. It is evident that, unlike the stressors, there are statistically significant differences in the application of stress coping methods across male and female professionals. Female professionals are more willing to seek external support and keep a positive attitude than males. This confirms Sunindijo and Kamardeen (2017) and Carr and Umberson (2013) who claimed that women tend to seek social support and use emotion-focussed coping strategies, such as distracting themselves and releasing their feelings more than men. Sunindijo and Kamardeen (2017) further asserted that female professionals were less represented in negative coping strategies such as alcohol, denial and escaping/distancing. On the contrary, the present study finds that female professionals adopt certain maladaptive coping methods more than males. These are: social isolation/escaping, emotional eating, blaming others, compulsive spending and releasing tension. Even in other maladaptive methods such as numbing and denial, females scored higher than males, and only in smoking did males score higher, though the p-values for these three methods are not significant. It appears that the gender plays a crucial role in stress coping styles.

The work stress model discussed in Figure 2.1 argues that the development of psychological strains is dependent on the stress coping methods adopted by individuals. A classification and regression tree was developed to investigate the interactions among work stress, stress coping methods and psychological strains. To streamline the investigation of the relationships, a single tree was developed by combining psychological outcomes such as burnout, anxiety and depression under one composite construct, psychological strains. Figure 2.9 presents the classification and regression tree for psychological strains and Table 2.11 shows the degree of influence of stress coping methods in predicting the outcomes. Five stress coping methods seem to be significant triggers of psychological strains among construction professionals, which are: blaming others, alcohol/drug consumption, releasing tension, emotional eating and drinking, and denial/distancing.

The CRT reveals some further information regarding the determinants of psychological strains and the interactions among them. Work stress is the primary trigger of psychological strains and the decision tree produced three groups of professionals based on the mean severity levels yielded for work stress: group 1

Table 2.11 Independent variable importance for psychological strains

Independent variable	Importance	Normalised importance
Work stress	.339	100.0%
Criticising or blaming others for the situation	.204	60.3%
Numbing – consuming alcohol or drugs to forget the stressful situation	.123	36.2%
Releasing tension by crying, yelling, throwing things, etc.	.099	29.2%
Emotional eating and drinking	.098	29.0%
Denial/distancing	.073	21.5%
Seeking external support	.053	15.7%
Resting and sleeping enough	.033	9.8%
Compulsive spending	.023	6.9%
Problem-solving	.023	6.7%
Physical activity (engaged in team sports, exercise, yoga or swimming)	.016	4.8%
Relaxation (mindfulness)	.014	4.2%
Escape – isolating from others	.014	4.1%
Engaged in humour, fun and leisure activities	.008	2.3%
Eating well-balanced meals	.007	1.9%
Smoking to get a relief from stress	.006	1.8%
Keeping a positive attitude	.006	1.8%
Gender	.002	.5%

Growing Method: CRT
Dependent Variable: Psychological strains

with mean values ≤.900, group 2 with mean values between .900 and 2.100, and group 3 with mean values ≥2.100. These can be classified as low, moderate and high levels of work stress. Around 11% of the professionals reported higher levels of work stress with a mean severity level of 2.235 on a scale ranging from 0 to 3, which alone contributes to psychological strains. Another 20% of them had the lowest stress level and the lowest psychological strains. For others, the combinations of work stress with different stress coping methods produce varying mental strain outcomes in the following manners:

• Those professionals who adopt active problem-solving and engage in humour and leisure activities have moderate psychological strains although their work stress severity levels are high; however, some others who combine active problem-solving (positive coping) with blaming others for the situation (negative coping), experience moderately high psychological strains.
• Professionals who experience moderate work stress but adopt a blaming style of coping reported moderately high psychological strains.
• Those who adopt a denial/distancing approach experience moderate mental strains although their stress level is low.

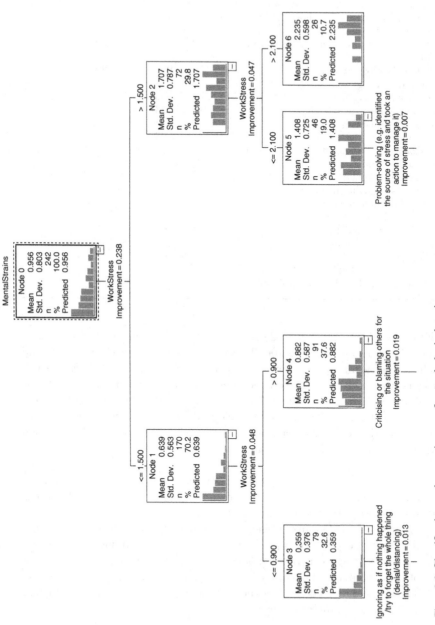

Figure 2.9 Classification and regression tree for psychological strains

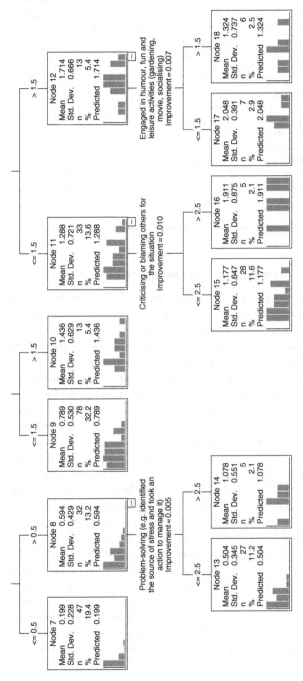

Figure 2.9 Continued

Table 2.12 Organisational interventions for stress management

Organisational intervention	Mean	S	Ranking
Implementing/improving polices and regulations on wellbeing and work conditions (workload, pay, career ladders, union involvement, work shifts, etc.)	.94	.879	2
Changing working conditions/organisational practices for better wellbeing of employees	.88	.855	3
Training employees to improve skills or job roles	1.03	.896	1
Training and educating supervisors and managers on wellbeing of subordinate staff	.79	.856	5
Training employees on stress management tactics	.60	.782	9
Facilitating access to relaxation or exercise programs	.65	.836	8
Promoting peer support groups	.68	.873	7
Providing psychological counselling/therapy programs	.83	1.019	4
Providing rehabilitation and return-to-work programs for wellbeing issues	.76	.978	6

Organisational interventions for stress management

The preceding section explored how coping methods adopted by individuals influence psychological strain outcomes in construction professionals. This section investigates the stress management interventions applied by organisations and their impact on stress, burnout, anxiety and depression. It also highlights the relationships between organisational interventions and job outcomes.

Table 2.12 presents the level of implementation of stress management interventions by organisations in the Australian construction industry. The overall level of implementation is low across the industry as evidenced by the mean ratings. For instance, the highest mean score yielded is 1.03 in the scale ranging from 0 to 3, and the others are lower than this.

Training employees to improve job skills is the mostly applied intervention, followed by changing work policies and then working conditions. Table 2.13 explains the results of Kruskal-Wallis H test to compare how the implementation of the interventions vary across different sizes of organisations. As revealed by the p-value of less than .05 for all the interventions, there is a statistically significant difference in the level of implementation across organisational sizes. Only large organisations with over 200 employees appear to implement interventions to a reasonable level, followed by medium sized organisations. Micro organisations are far below other size categories except for promoting peer support groups. Given that most micro organisations in the construction industry are sole-traders or partnerships between a few people, other intervention methods may be less relevant and/or costly to them. They seem to rely on peer mentoring arrangements facilitated by Safe Work Australia and professional institutions that they belong to.

Table 2.13 Stress interventions by the organisation size

Intervention	Organisation size	N	Mean rank	Kruskal-Wallis H	Sig.
Implementing/improving polices and regulations on wellbeing and work conditions (workload, pay, career ladders, union involvement, work shifts, etc.)	employees ≤4	20	81.25	19.360	.000
	5 to 19 employees	40	96.01		
	20 to 199 employees	71	103.73		
	employees ≥200	92	132.02		
Changing working conditions/ organisational practices for better wellbeing of employees	employees ≤4	20	89.18	13.085	.000
	5 to 19 employees	40	94.36		
	20 to 199 employees	71	107.96		
	employees ≥200	92	127.74		
Training employees to improve skills or job roles	employees ≤4	20	86.60	14.479	.002
	5 to 19 employees	41	102.71		
	20 to 199 employees	71	102.30		
	employees ≥200	92	130.36		
Training and educating supervisors and managers on wellbeing of subordinate staff	employees ≤4	20	92.63	8.476	.037
	5 to 19 employees	39	101.31		
	20 to 199 employees	71	105.23		
	employees ≥200	92	124.76		
Training employees on stress management tactics	employees ≤4	20	94.95	22.944	.000
	5 to 19 employees	38	89.22		
	20 to 199 employees	71	99.41		
	employees ≥200	92	132.43		
Facilitating access to relaxation or exercise programs	employees ≤4	20	88.75	31.975	.000
	5 to 19 employees	38	81.68		
	20 to 199 employees	71	100.96		
	employees ≥200	92	135.70		
Promoting peer support groups	employees ≤4	20	117.18	16.135	.001
	5 to 19 employees	38	86.96		
	20 to 199 employees	71	101.09		
	employees ≥200	92	127.23		
Providing psychological counselling/ therapy programs	employees ≤4	20	83.73	46.456	.000
	5 to 19 employees	38	71.54		
	20 to 199 employees	71	101.39		
	employees ≥200	92	140.64		
Providing rehabilitation and return-to-work programs for wellbeing issues	employees ≤4	20	71.43	34.433	.000
	5 to 19 employees	38	88.82		
	20 to 199 employees	71	100.20		
	employees ≥200	91	136.18		

Table 2.14 illustrates the correlations between organisational stress interventions and psychological strains and job outcomes among construction industry professionals. The correlation coefficient for a given association can range from −1.0 to +1.0 with (−) sign denoting a negative correlation and (+) sign for a positive correlation between the concerned variables. The strength of the correlation is determined by the coefficient value. Nardi (2014) suggested that coefficients below .30 are considered weak, those between .30 to .70 are moderate and those above .70 are strong. The interventions have statistically significant negative correlations with psychological strains such as work stress, burnout,

Table 2.14 Correlations between interventions, and psychological strains and job outcomes

Interventions	Psychological strains and job outcomes					
	Work stress	Burnout	Anxiety	Depression	Job satisfaction	Job performance
Implementing/improving polices and regulations on wellbeing and work conditions (workload, pay, career ladders, union involvement, work shifts, etc.)	-.186**	-.208**	-.202**	-.194**	.347**	.117
Changing working conditions/organisational practices for better wellbeing of employees	-.293**	-.310**	-.206**	-.185**	.407**	.183**
Training employees to improve skills or job roles	-.217**	-.240**	-.169*	-.122	.420**	.172*
Training and educating supervisors and managers on wellbeing of subordinate staff	-.251**	-.279**	-.162*	-.120	.414**	.105
Training employees on stress management tactics	-.230**	-.240**	-.149*	-.119	.338**	.147*
Facilitating access to relaxation or exercise programs	-.198**	-.216**	-.170*	-.166*	.264**	.113
Promoting peer support groups	-.219**	-.194**	-.080	-.062	.370**	.135*
Providing psychological counselling/therapy programs	-.093	-.132*	-.025	-.014	.239**	.104
Providing rehabilitation and return-to-work programs for wellbeing issues	-.113	-.197**	-.077	-.045	.296**	.137*

** Correlation is significant at the .01 level (2-tailed).
* Correlation is significant at the .05 level (2-tailed).

anxiety and depression. However, the strengths of correlations are in the weak range. Statistically significant positive correlations are discernible between the interventions and job satisfaction, and the strengths of the correlations are moderate. Similarly, the interventions appear to have statistically significant positive correlations with job performance, but the strength of association is weak. These findings partially support the stress model shown in Figure 2.1 about the role of organisational interventions in minimising work stress and its consequences.

Conclusion

The present study reveals that around 90% of construction professionals in Australia endure work stress and burnout due to work stress. Similarly, work stress induced anxiety and depression are as high as around 60% and 50%, respectively, with around 15% suffering from severe burnout, anxiety and depression. Within this cohort, female professionals experience more severe anxiety and depression than their counterpart. Work–life conflict is the prime contributor of work stress, which is mediated by unpredictable work hours and excessive workload. Negative effects of these stressors are, however, subdued by the presence of career progression opportunities, satisfactory salaries, job security and consultation culture at work. Similarly, professionals who deploy coping strategies such as thoughtful problem-solving and leisure and fun activities with socialisation manage the stress well. While a considerable proportion of individuals adopt a range of positive coping methods, a large portion of organisations in the construction industry implement stress control interventions only at a minimum level – only tertiary interventions, except for large organisations with over 200 employees. Employees of organisations that implement primary and secondary interventions experience lower work stress, burnout, anxiety and depression as well as have higher job satisfaction.

In light of these findings, the following are suggested to improve the condition in the construction industry:

- Organisations of all sizes and types in the construction industry should consider implementing flexible work and homeworking arrangements as practical as possible to arrest stress caused by work–life conflict.
- Employments in the construction industry should feature opportunities for career development, competitive salaries and job security to counteract work stress.
- Nurturing strong supportive and consultation culture is crucial to minimise work stress and its negative effects.
- Individual professionals should maintain a healthy lifestyle enriched with a balanced diet, regular physical activity and leisure socialisation and fun. At work, they should engage in an adequate level of consultation and communications with colleagues regularly to actively resolve stressors.
- Small and medium organisations in the construction industry should regard the implementation of primary and secondary stress intervention measures as investments for achieving productivity enhancements.

All in all, the construction industry is unique from many other sectors and it is one of the worst industries for work stress and related psychological disorders. This situation not only affects individual professionals and their families, but also construction organisations. There are specific ways that stressors manifest and solutions therefore need to be tailored to suit the culture and operations of the industry. Concerted efforts from individual professionals, organisations, industry bodies and the government/policy makers are required to achieve a socially sustainable construction industry.

References

Ajayi, S.O. (2018). Effect of stress on employee performance and job satisfaction: a case study of Nigerian banking industry. *Labor: Personnel Economics eJournal*. DOI: 10.2139/ssrn.3160620.

Akgunduz Y. (2013). The influence of self-esteem and role stress on job performance in hotel businesses. *International Journal of Contemporary Hospitality Management, 27*(6), 1082–1099.

Al-Maskari, F., Shah, S.M., Al-Sharhan, R., Al-Haj, E., Al-Kaabi, K., Khonji, D., Schneider, J.D., Nagelkerke, N.J. and Bernsen, R.M. (2011). Prevalence of depression and suicidal behaviors among male migrant workers in United Arab Emirates. *Journal of Immigrant and Minority Health, 13*(6), 1027–1032. https://doi.org/10.1007/s10903-011-9470-9.

Amato, P.R. (2015). Marriage, cohabitation and mental health. *Family Matters, 96*, 5–13.

Anxiety and Depression Association of America (ADAA). (2018). Generalised Anxiety Disorder. Retrieved 18 June, 2020, from https://adaa.org/understanding-anxiety/generalized-anxiety-disorder-gad.

Applebaum, D., Fowler, S., Fiedler, N., Osinubi, O. and Robson, M. (2010). The impact of environmental factors on nursing stress, job satisfaction, and turnover intention. *Journal of Nursing Administration, 40*(7/8), 323–328.

Arditi, D., Gluch, P. and Holmdahl, M. (2013). Managerial competencies of female and male managers in the Swedish construction industry. *Construction Management and Economics, 31*(9), 979–990. DOI:10.1080/01446193.2013.828845.

Beyond Blue. (2020). Depression. Retrieved 13 February, 2020, from www.beyondblue.org.au/the-facts/depression.

Black Dog Institute. (2018). Trauma and mental health. Retrieved 6 January, 2020, from https://blackdoginstitute.org.au/research/key-research-areas/trauma-and-mental-health.

Blanch, A. (2016). Social support as a mediator between job control and psychological strain. *Social Science & Medicine, 157*, 148–155. doi:10.1016/j.socscimed.2016.04.007.

Boschman, J.S., van der Molen, H.F., Sluiter, J.K. and Frings-Dresen, M.H. (2013). Psychosocial work environment and mental health among construction workers. *Applied Ergonomics, 44*(5), 748–755. https://doi.org/10.1016/j.apergo.2013.01.004.

Bowen, P., Edwards, P. and Lingard, H. (2013). Workplace stress experienced by construction professionals in South Africa. *Journal of Construction Engineering and Management, 139*(4), 393–403.

Bowen, P., Govender, R. and Edwards, P. (2014). Structural equation modeling of occupational stress in the construction industry. *Journal of Construction Engineering and Management, 140*(9), 04014042. https://doi.org/10.1061/(ASCE)CO.1943-7862.0000877.

Bowen, P., Govender, R., Edwards, P. and Cattell, K. (2018). Work-related contact, work-family conflict, psychological distress, and sleep problems experienced by construction professionals: an integrated explanatory model. *Construction Management and Economics*, *36*(3), 153–174. https://doi.org/10.1080/01446193.2017.1341638.

Braverman, M. (1992). Posttrauma crisis intervention in the workplace. In J.C. Quick, L.R. Murphy and J.J. Hurrell, Jr. (Eds.), *Stress & Well-Being at Work: Assessments and Interventions for Occupational Mental Health* (pp299–316). American Psychological Association. https://doi.org/10.1037/10116-020.

Brotheridge, C.M. and Grandey, A.A. (2002). Emotional labor and burnout: comparing two perspectives of "people work". *Journal of Vocational Behavior, 60*(1), 17–39. https://doi.org/10.1006/jvbe.2001.1815.

Carr, D., and Umberson, D. (2013). The social psychology of stress, health, and coping. In J. DeLamater and A. Ward (Eds.), *Handbook of Social Psychology*, 2nd Ed. Dordrecht, Netherlands: Springer.

Carver, C.S., Scheier, M.F. and Weintraub, J.K. (1989). Assessing coping strategies: a theoretically based approach. *J. Personality Social Psychol., 56*(2), 267–283.

Cattell, K., Bowen, P. and Edwards, P. (2016). Stress among South African construction professionals: a job demand-control-support survey. *Construction Management and Economics, 34*(10), 700–723.

Chan, A.P.C., Nwaogu, J.M. and Naslund, J.A. (2020). Mental ill-health risk factors in the construction industry: systematics review. *Journal of Construction Engineering and Management, 146*(3), 04020004.

Chang, E.M., Daly, J., Haancock, K.M., Bidewell, J.W., Johnson, A., Lambert, V.A. and Lambert, C.E. (2006). The relationships among workplace stressors, coping methods, demographic characteristics, and health in Australian nurses. *Journal of Professional Nursing, 22*(1), 30–38.

Chartered Institute of Building (CIOB). (2006). Occupational stress in the construction industry. Retrieved 30 January, 2020, from https://policy.ciob.org/wp-content/uploads/2006/03/Occupational-Stress-in-the-Construction-Industry-March-2006.pdf.

Clarke, S. and Cooper, C. (2004). *Managing the Risk of Workplace Stress*. London: Routledge. https://doi.org/10.4324/9780203644362.

Collins, S. (2008). Statutory social workers: stress, job satisfaction, coping, social support and individual differences. *British Journal of Social Work – BRIT J SOC WORK, 38*, 1173–1193. 10.1093/bjsw/bcm047.

Cooper, C.L., Dewe, P.J. and O'Driscoll, M.P. (2001). *Organizational Stress: A New Critique of Theory, Research and Applications*. Thousand Oaks, SA: Sage.

Dainty, A.R. and Lingard, H. (2006). Indirect discrimination in construction organizations and the impact on women's careers. *Journal of Management in Engineering, 22*(3), 108–118. 10.1061/(ASCE)0742-597X(2006).

Day, A.L. and Livingstone, H. (2001). Chronic and acute stressors among military personnel: do coping styles buffer their negative impact on health? *Journal of Occupational Health Psychology, 6*(4), 348–360.

de Jonge, J., Bosma, H., Peter, R. and Siegrist, J. (2000). Job strain, effort-reward imbalance and employee well-being: a large-scale cross-sectional study. *Social Science and Medicine, 50*(9), 1317–1327.

Demsky, C.A. (2012). Interpersonal conflict and employee well-being: the moderating role of recovery experiences. Dissertations and Theses. Paper 766. doi:10.15760/etd.766.

Ducharme, L.J and Martin, J.K. (2000). Unrewarding work, coworker support and job satisfaction: a test of the buffering hypothesis. *Work and Occupation, 27*(2), 223–243.

Evans, G.W., Johansson, G. and Carrere, S. (1994). Psychosocial factors and the physical environment: inter-relations in the workplace. In C.L. Cooper and I.T. Robertson (Eds.), *International Review of Industrial and Organizational Psychology*. Chichester, UK: Wiley.

Felmingham, K.L., Tran, T.P., Fong, W.C. and Bryant, R.A. (2012). Sex differences in emotional memory consolidation: the effect of stress induced salivary alpha-amylase and cortisol. *Biological Psychology, 89*(3), 539–544.

Foster, A.D. (2014). Traumatic life events and symptoms of anxiety: moderating effects of adaptive versus maladaptove coping strategies. Unpublished thesis, University of East Tennessee State University. Retrieved 11 February, 2020, from https://dc.etsu.edu/cgi/viewcontent.cgi?article=3741&context=etd.

Friedman, M. and Rosenman, R. (1974). *Type A Behavior and Your Heart*. New York, NY: Random House.

Friedman, M. and Rosenman, R.H. (1959). Association of specific overt behaviour pattern with blood and cardiovascular findings. *Journal of American Medical Association, 169*(12), 1286–1296.

Frone, M.R. (2000). Interpersonal conflict at work and psychological outcomes: testing a model among young workers. *Journal of Occupational Health Psychology, 5*(2), 246–255. https://doi.org/10.1037/1076-8998.5.2.246.

Fryers, T., Melzer, D. and Jenkins, R. (2003). Social inequalities and the common mental disorders: a systematic review of the evidence. *Social Psychiatry and Psychiatric Epidemiology, 38*(5), 229–237.

Glozier, N. (2017). Review of evidence of psychological risks for mental ill-health in the workplace. Retrieved 18 June, 2020, from https://esf.com.au/wp-content/uploads/2020/05/Glozier-Review-of-Evidence-of-Psychosocial-Risks-for-Mental-.._.pdf.

Goldsmith, E. (2007). Stress, fatigue, and social support in the work and family context. *Journal of Loss and Trauma, 12*(2), 155–169. https://doi.org/10.1080/15434610600854228.

Hallberg, U.E., Johansson, G. and Schaufeli, W.B. (2007). Type A behavior and work situation: Associations with burnout and work engagement. *Scandinavian Journal of Psychology, 48*(2), 135–142.

Harvey, S.B., Modini, M., Joyce, S., Milligan-Saville, J.S., Leona Tan, L., Mykletun, A., Bryant, R.A., Christensen, H. and Mitchell, P.B. (2017). Can work make you mentally ill? A systematic meta-review of work-related risk factors for common mental health problems. *Occupational and Environmental Medicine, 74*(4), 301–310.

Health and Safety Executive (HSE). (2019). Tackling work-related stress using the management standards approach. Retrieved 30 January, 2020, from www.hse.gov.uk/pubns/wbk01.pdf.

Howard, K., Giblin, M. and Medina, R. (2018). The relationship between occupational stress and gastrointestinal illness: a comprehensive study of public school teachers. *Journal of Workplace Behavioral Health, 33*(3–4), 260–275.

Hu, B.S., Liang, Y.X., Hu, X.Y., Long, Y.F. and Ge, L.N. (2013). Posttraumatic stress disorder in co-workers following exposure to a fatal construction accident in China. *International Journal of Occupational and Environmental Health, 6*(3), 203–207. https://doi.org/10.1179/oeh.2000.6.3.203.

IBM Corporation. (2012). IBM SPSS Decision Trees 21. Retrieved 10 February, 2020, from www.sussex.ac.uk/its/pdfs/SPSS_Decision_Trees_21.pdf.

Jacobsen, H.B., Caban-Martinez, A., Onyebeke, L.C., Sorensen, G., Dennerlein, J.T. and Reme, S.E. (2013). Construction workers struggle with a high prevalence of mental distress, and this is associated with their pain and injuries. *J. Occup. Environ. Med.*, *55*(10), 1197–1204. https://doi.org/10.1097/JOM.0b013e31829c76b3.

Jamal, M. (1999). Job stress, type-A behavior, and well-being: A cross-cultural examination. *International Journal of Stress Management*, *6*(1), 57–67.

Jeung, D., Kim, C. and Chang, S. (2018). Emotional labor and burnout: a review of the literature. *Yonsei Medical Journal*, *59*(2), 187–193.

Jex, S.M. (1998). *Advanced Topics in Organizational Behavior. Stress and Job Performance: Theory, Research, and Implications for Managerial Practice.* Sage Publications Ltd.

Jick, T.D. and Mitz, L.F. (1985). Sex differences in work stress. *The Academy of Management Review*, *10*(3), 408–420.

Kamardeen, I. (2020). *Preventing Workplace Incidents in Construction*. London: Routledge https://doi.org/10.1201/9781315110462.

Kamardeen, I. and Sunindijo, R.Y. (2017). Personal characteristics moderate work stress in construction professionals. *Journal Construction Engineering and Management*, *143*(10), 04017072. https://doi.org/10.1061/(ASCE)CO.1943-7862.0001386.

Kanayo, D.O. (2016). The influence of self-esteem and role stress on job performance of technical college employees. *International Journal of Online and Distance Learning*, *1*(1), 58–75.

Keegel, T., Ostry, A. and LaMontagne, A. (2009). Job strain exposures vs. stress-related workers compensation claims in Victoria, Australia: developing a public health response to job stress. *Journal of Public Health Policy*, *30*(1), 17–39. 10.1057/jphp.2008.41.

Kessler, R.C., Berglund, P., Demler, O., Jin, R., Merikangas, K.R. and Walters, E.E. (2005). Lifetime prevalence and age-of-onset distributions of DSM-IV disorders in the national comorbidity survey replication. *Archives of General Psychiatry*, *62*(6), 593–602.

Kobasa, S.C., Maddi, S.R. and Kahn, S. (1982). Hardiness and health: a prospective study. *Journal of Personality and Social Psychology*, *42*(1), 168–177. https://doi.org/10.1037/0022-3514.42.1.168.

Landy, F.J. and Conte, J.M. (2006). *Work in the 21st Century: An Introduction to Industrial and Organizational Psychology*, 2nd ed. Malden, USA: Wiley-Blackwell.

Leather, P., Pygras, M., Beale, D. and Lawrence, C. (1998). Windows in the workplace: sunlight, view and occupational stress. *Environment and Behavior*, *30*(6), 739–762.

Leavy, R.L. (1983). Social support and psychological disorder: a review. *Journal of Community Psychology*, *11*(1), 3–21

Leka, S.L., Griffiths, A. and Cox, T. (2003). *Work Organization and Stress: Systematic Problem Approaches for Employers, Manages and Trade Union Representatives*. Geneva: World Health Organization.

Leung, M., Chan, I.Y.S. and Cooper, C.L. (2015). Stress Management in the Construction Industry. Chichester, UK: Wiley Blackwell.

Leung, M., Chan, Y.S.I. and Dongyu, C. (2011). Structural linear relationships between job stress, burnout, physiological stress, and performance of construction project managers. *Engineering, Construction and Architectural Management*, *18*(3), 312–328.

Leung, M-Y., Chan, Y-S. and Yuen, K-W. (2010). Impacts of stressors and stress on the injury incidents of construction workers in Hong Kong. *Journal of Construction Engineering and Management*, *136*(10), 1093–1103.

Levy, P.E. (2010). *Industrial/ Organizational Psychology*, 3rd ed. New York: Worth Publishers.

Lim, S., Chi, S., Lee, J.D., Lee, H.J. and Choi, H. (2018). Analyzing psychological conditions of field-workers in the construction industry. *International Journal of Occupational and Environmental Health*, *23*(4), 261–281. https://doi.org/10.1080/10773525.2018.1474419.

Lingard, H. and Francis, V. (2004). The work-life experiences of office and site-based employees in the Australian construction industry. *Construction Management & Economics*, *22*, 991–1002. 10.1080/0144619042000241444.

Lingard, H. and Francis, V. (2006). Does a supportive work environment moderate the relationship between work-family conflict and burnout among construction professionals? *Construction Management and Economics*, *24*(2), 185–196.

Lingard, H. and Francis, V. (2009). *Managing Work-Life Balance in Construction*. London: Taylor & Francis Group.

Lingard, H., Brown, K., Bradley, L., Bailey, C. and Townsend, K. (2007). Improving employees' work-life balance in the construction industry: project alliance case study. *Journal of Construction Engineering and Management*, *133*(10), 807–815. https://doi.org/10.1061/(ASCE)0733-9364(2007)133:10(807).

Loosemore, M. and Waters, T. (2004). Gender differences in occupational stress among professionals in the construction industry. *Journal of Management in Engineering*, *3*(126), 126–132. 10.1061/(ASCE)0742-597X(2004)20.

Love, P.E., Edwards, D.J. and Irani, Z. (2010). Work stress, support, and mental health in construction. *J. Constr. Eng. Manage*, *136*(6), 650–658. https://doi.org/10.1061/(ASCE) CO.1943-7862.0000165.

Lundberg, U. and Frankenhaeuser, M. (1999). Stress and workload of men and women in high-ranking positions. *Journal of Occupational Health Psychology*, *4*(2), 142–151. https://doi.org/10.1037/1076-8998.4.2.142.

Mann, S. (2004). People-work: emotion management, stress and coping. *British Journal of Guid Counc*, *32*, 205–221.

Mayo Clinic. (2018). Anxiety disorders. Retrieved 20 February, 2020, from www.mayoclinic.org/diseases-conditions/anxiety/symptoms-causes/syc-20350961#:~:text=Common%20anxiety%20signs%20and%20symptoms,Having%20an%20increased%20heart%20rate.

McCoy, J.M. (2002). Work environment. In R.B. Bechtel and A. Churchman (Eds.), *Handbook of Environmental Psychology*. New York: John Wiley & Sons.

Michie, S. (2002). Causes and management of stress at work. *Occupational and Environmental Medicine*, *59*(1), 67–72. https://doi.org/10.1136/oem.59.1.67.

Muchinsky, P.M. (2006). *Psychology Applied to Work: An Introduction to Industrial and Organizational Psychology*. Belmont, CA: Thomson/Wadsworth.

Mueller, D. (1980). Social networks: a promising direction for research on the relationship of the social environment to psychiatric disorder. *Social Science and Medicine*, *14*(2), 147–161.

Nardi, P.M. (2014). *Doing Survey Research: A Guide to Quantitative Methods*, 3rd Ed. Boulder; London: Paradigm Publishers.

Ndjaboué, R., Brisson, C. and Vézina, M. (2012). Organisational justice and mental health: a systematic review of prospective studies. *Occup Environ Med*, *69*(10), 694–700. doi:10.1136/oemed-2011-100595.

Niedhammer, I., Chastang, J.F., Gendrey, L., David, S. and Degioanni, S. (2006). [Psychometric properties of the French version of Karasek's 'Job Content Questionnaire' and its scales measuring psychological demands, decision latitude and social support: the results of the SUMER survey]. *Sante Publique*, *18*(3), 413–427.

Nieuwenhuijsen, K., Bruinvels, D. and Frings-Dresen, M. (2010). Psychosocial work environment and stress-related disorders, a systematic review. *Occupational Medicine*, *60*(2), 277–286.

Nwaogu, J., Chan, A.P.C., Hon, C.K.H. and Darko, A. (2019). Review of global mental health research in the construction industry: A science mapping approach. *Engineering Construction & Architectural Management.* ahead-of-print. 10.1108/ECAM-02-2019-0114.

Olofsdotter, G. and Randevåg, L. (2016). Doing masculinities in construction project management: we understand each other, but she. *Gender in Manage: An International Journal, 31*(2), 134–153.

Park, J. and Jung, M. (2009). A note on determination of sample size for a Likert scale. *Communications of the Korean Statistical Society, 16*(4), 669–673.

Paunio, T., Korhonen, T., Hublin, C., Partinen, M., Koskenvuo, K., Koskenvuo, M. and Kaprio, J. (2015). Poor sleep predicts symptoms of depression and disability retirement due to depression. *Journal of Affective Disorders, 172*, 381–389.

Phillip, K. (2019). Six ways your office can reduce stress. Retrieved 20 July, 2019, from www.morganlovell.co.uk/knowledge/opinion-pieces/six-ways-your-office-can-reduce-stress/.

Pugliesi, K. and Shook, S.L. (1997). Gender, jobs, and emotional labor in a complex organization. In R.J. Erickson and B. Cuthbertson-Johnson (Eds.), *Social Perspectives on Emotion* (Vol. 4), pp283–316. New York: JAI.

Quick, J., Wright, T., Adkins, J., Nelson, D. and Quick, J. (2013). *Preventive Stress Management in Organizations*, 2nd ed. Washington: APA Publishing. 10.1037/13942-000.

Raffaello, M. and Maass, A. (2002). Chronic exposure to noise in industry: the effects on satisfaction, stress symptoms and company attachment. *Environment and Behavior, 34*(5), 651–671.

Ramaswami, M. and Bhaskaran, R. (2010). A CHAID based performance prediction model in educational data mining. *International Journal of Computer Science Issues, 7*(1), 10–18.

Robbins, S.P., Bergman, R., Stagg, I. and Coulter, M. (2015). *Management*, 7th ed. Melbourne, Australia: Pearson Australia.

Roche, A., Lee, N.K., Battams, S., Fischer, J.A., Cameron, J. and McEntee, A. (2015). Alcohol use among workers in male-dominated industries: a systematic review of risk factors. *Safety Science, 78*, 124–141. DOI: 10.1016/j.ssci.2015.04.007.

Roquelaure, Y. (2018). Musculoskeletal disorders and psychosocial factors at work. ETUI Research Paper – Report 142. Available at SSRN. Retrieved 12 November, 2019, from https://ssrn.com/abstract=3316143 or http://dx.doi.org/10.2139/ssrn.3316143.

Ross, R.J., Ball, W.A., Sullivan, K.A. and Caroff, S.N. (1989). Sleep disturbance as the hallmark of posttraumatic stress disorder. *American Journal of Psychiatry, 146*(6), 697–707. doi:10.1176/ajp.146.6.697.

Rossi, A.M., Quick, J.C. and Perrewe, P.L. (2009). *Stress and Quality of Working Life: The Positive and the Negative.* Information Age Pub.

Sabel, B.A., Wang, J., Cárdenas-Morales, L., Faiq, M. and Heim, C. (2018). Mental stress as consequence and cause of vision loss: the dawn of psychosomatic ophthalmology for preventive and personalized medicine. *EPMA J, 9*(2), 133–160. doi:10.1007/s13167-018-0136-8.

Safe Work Australia. (2006). Work-related mental disorders in Australia. Retrieved 4 February, 2020, from www.safeworkaustralia.gov.au/doc/work-related-mental-disorders-australia.

Safe Work Australia. (2016). Guide for preventing and responding to workplace bullying. Retrieved 10 June, 2020, from www.safeworkaustralia.gov.au/system/files/documents/1702/guide-preventing-responding-workplace-bullying.pdf/.

Safe Work Australia. (2018). Supporting business to provide a mentally healthy workplace. Retrieved 4 February, 2020, from www.safeworkaustralia.gov.au/book/supporting-business-provide-mentally-healthy-workplace.

Safe Work Australia. (2019). Work-related psychological health and safety: A systematic approach to meeting your duties. Retrieved 3 March, 2020, from www.safeworkaustralia. gov.au/system/files/documents/1911/work-related_psychological_health_and_ safety_a_systematic_approach_to_meeting_your_duties.pdf.

Safe Work Australia. (n.d.). Mental health. Retrieved 18 June, 2020, from www. safeworkaustralia.gov.au/topic/mental-health.

Salvagioni, D.A.J., Melanda, F.N., Mesas, A.E., González, A.D., Gabani, F.L. and Andrade, S.M.D. (2017). Physical, psychological and occupational consequences of job burnout: a systematic review of prospective studies. *PLoS ONE*, *12*(10): e0185781. https://doi.org/ 10.1371/journal.pone.0185781.

Sara, J.D., Prasad, M., Eleid, M.F., Zhang, M., Widmer, R.J. and Lerman, A. (2018). Association between work-related stress and coronary heart disease: a review of prospective studies through the job strain, effort-reward balance, and organizational justice models. *Journal of the American Heart Association*, *7*(9), e008073. https://doi.org/10.1161/ JAHA.117.008073.

Schmidt, S., Roesler, U., Kusserow, T. and Rau, R. (2014). Uncertainty in the workplace: examining role ambiguity and role conflict, and their link to depression-a meta-analysis. *European Journal of Work and Organizational Psychology*, *23*(1), 91–106. 10.1080/ 1359432X.2012.711523.

Shea, T., Pettit, T. and Cieri, H.D. (2011). Work environment stress: the impact of the physical work environment on psychological health. Monash University. Retrieved 23 November, 2020, from http://research.iscrr.com.au/__data/assets/pdf_file/0007/ 297763/Work-environment-stress-impact-on-psychological-health.pdf.

Skogstad, M., Skorstad, M., Lie, A., Conradi, H.S., Heir, T. and Weisæth, L. (2013). Work-related post-traumatic stress disorder. *Occupational Medicine*, *63*(3), 175–182.

Song, Y. and Lu, Y. (2015). Decision tree methods: applications for classification and prediction. *Shanghai Archives of Psychiatry*, *27*(2), 130–135. 10.11919/j.issn.1002-0829.215044.

Spector, P.E. and Jex, S. (1998). Development of four self-report measures of job stressors and strain: interpersonal conflict at work scale, organizational constraints scale, quantitative workload inventory, and physical symptoms inventory. *Journal of Occupational Health Psychology*, *3*, 356–367.

Sunindijo, R.Y. and Kamardeen, I. (2017). Work stress is a threat to gender diversity in the construction industry. *J. Constr. Eng. Manage*, *143*(10), 04017073. https://doi.org/ 10.1061/(ASCE)CO.1943-7862.0001387.

Suteeraroj, M. and Ussahawanitchakit, P. (2008). Stress, anxiety, and intention to leave: the empirical study of managers in Thai petroleum and chemical businesses. *Review of Business Research*, *8*(4), 163–173.

Sutherland, V. and Davidson, M.J. (1993). Using a stress audit: the construction site manager experience in the UK. *Work Stress*, *7*(3), 273–286. https://doi.org/10.1080/ 02678379308257067.

Tavakol, M. and Dennick, R. (2011). Making sense of Cronbach's alpha. *International Journal of Medical Education*, *2*, 53–55. https://doi.org/10.5116/ijme.4dfb.8dfd.

The American Institute of Stress. (2019). 42 worrying workplace stress statistics. Retrieved 30 January, 2020, from www.stress.org/42-worrying-workplace-stress-statistics.

Theorell, T., Hammarström, A., Aronsson, G., Bendz, L., Grape, T., Hogstedt, C., Marteinsdottir, I., Skoog, I. and Hall, C. (2015). A systematic review including meta-analysis of work environment and depressive symptoms. *BMC Public Health*, *15*(1). 10.1186/s12889-015-1954-4.

Thoits, P.A. (2010). Stress and health: major findings and policy implications. *Journal of Health Social Behaviour*, *51*(1), S41–S53.

Tomiyama, A. (2019). Stress and obesity. *Annual Review of Psychology*, 703–718.

Verkuil, B., Atasayi, S. and Molendijk, M.L. (2015). Workplace bullying and mental health: a meta-analysis on cross-sectional and longitudinal data. *PLoS ONE, 10*(8), e0135225. https://doi.org/10.1371/journal.pone.0135225.

VicHealth. (2012). *Reducing Stress in the Workplace (An Evidence Review: Summary Report)*. Victorian Health Promotion Foundation, Melbourne, Australia.

Viswesvaran, C., Sanchez, J.I. and Fisher, J. (1999). The role of social support in the process of work stress: a meta-analysis. *Journal of Vocational Behavior, 54*(2), 314–334.

Wang, H. (2018). The impact of social support on work stress and job burnout. 10.13140/RG.2.2.27371.44323.

Weinberg, R.S. and Gould, D. (2011). *Foundations of Sport and Exercise Psychology*, 5th Ed. Champaign, IL: Human Kinetics.

Wickens, C.D. and Hollands, J.G. (2000). Engineering Psychology and Human Performance, 3rd Ed. Upper Saddle River, NJ: Prentice Hall.

World Health Organization (WHO). (2019). Burn-out an occupational phenomenon: international classification of diseases. Retrieved 13 February, 2020, from www.who.int/mental_health/evidence/burn-out/en/.

Zapf, D. (2002). Emotion work and psychological well-being: a review of the literature and some conceptual considerations. *Human Resource Management Review, 12*, 237–268.

3 Work stress induced chronic insomnia in construction

Adequate, quality sleep is an essential human need that provides natural restoration for the central nervous and the physiological systems of the body. It directly affects the mental and physical health and performance, including brain and heart health, immune system, metabolism, emotional balance, productivity, attention, memory and learning, creativity and vitality. Recent epidemiological research revealed that sleep quality and quantity has been declining and the symptoms of insomnia have become more rampant among the working population during the past three decades due to long work hours, shift work and work stress that is triggered by poor psychosocial work characteristics (Härmä 2013; Paunio, Tuisku and Korhonen 2015). It is evident that there is a bi-directional relationship between work stress and sleep, forming a vicious cycle, i.e. work stress affects an individual's sleep, which in turn affects work performance, leading to more work stress (Swanson et al. 2011).

A plethora of recent research concluded that construction professionals endure chronic work stress, which suggests that they may be suffering from chronic insomnia and its consequences in physiological, psychological and job performance dimensions. However, this is an underexplored topic in the construction literature. Hence, this chapter investigates work stress induced insomnia among construction professionals in Australia and its subsequent impacts on their physical and psychological health as well as job outcomes.

The chapter is organised as follows. First, definitions of insomnia and its general causes and effects are provided, followed by a discussion on work-related risk factors for chronic insomnia. Then, explanations of the research method applied to study the construction context are provided. Next, findings of the data analytics around the prevalence of work stress induced chronic insomnia among construction professionals, influence of factors such as job role, gender and age on insomnia occurrences and association between chronic insomnia and other medical complications in construction professionals are elaborated on. Finally, concluding insights are drawn for the construction industry.

Healthy sleep

Healthy sleep is as essential to survival as healthy food and clean water to humans. It plays a critical role in the health and wellbeing as well as for brain functioning.

Table 3.1 Recommended sleep hours

Age	Required sleep
Newborn (0–3 months)	14–17 hrs
Infant (4–11 months)	12–15 hrs
Toddler (1–2 years)	11–14 hrs
Pre-schooler (3–5 years)	10–13 hrs
School-age child (6–13 years)	9–11 hrs
Teen (14–17 years)	8–10 hrs
Young adult (18–25 years)	7–9 hrs
Adult (26–64 years)	7–9 hrs
Older adult (65+ years)	7–8 hrs

Source: American Psychiatric Association (2019)

A good night's sleep helps recover physically and psychologically by: (1) restoring energy resources of the body, (2) allowing organs to rest and recover, (3) removing toxins from the brain that accumulate during waking hours, (4) boosting the immune system and healing process, and (5) restoring cognitive, learning and memory processes and functions (Åkerstedt and Nilsson 2003; Paunio, Tuisku and Korhonen 2015). A healthy sleep is achieved by getting an adequate quantity of quality sleep at the right times, generally at night. National Sleep Foundation (2019) defined quality sleep as being when one is able to fall asleep within 30 minutes, sleep soundly throughout the night with no more than one awakening, and fall back asleep within 20 minutes after wakening. To the contrary, poor sleep is characterised by trouble falling and staying asleep, restlessness and early wakening. The required hours of quality sleep per day varies with age, as shown in Table 3.1.

Sleep disorders, on the other hand, occur due to problems with the quantity, quality and timing of sleep. Different types of sleep disorders exist, namely insomnia, narcolepsy, obstructive sleep apnea and restless leg syndrome, of which insomnia is the most prevalent (American Psychiatric Association 2019). There is increasing evidence from western countries for a high prevalence of insomnia. For instance, Sutton, Moldofsky and Badley (2001), and Hossain and Shapiro (2002) reported that around one-fifth of the Canadian general population endure insomnia. Moreover, Härmä (2013) and Paunio, Tuisku and Korhonen (2015) posited that insomnia has become widespread among the working population over the past three decades.

Insomnia

Insomnia refers to the inability to obtain adequate, quality sleep and is characterised by the following symptoms (Riba 1993):

- sleep onset insomnia (difficulty falling asleep)
- interrupted sleep characterised by frequent wakening during the night and having difficulty to fall back asleep

- waking up too early in the morning and not being able to fall back asleep
- feeling daytime fatigue.

WebMD (2019) categorised insomnia into two types, acute or chronic. Acute insomnia is short and can last from one night to a few weeks whereas chronic insomnia can last long, with a person having insomnia three or more nights a week over three months or longer. Acute insomnia is usually caused by major life changes/losses (job loss or change, loss of loved ones, divorce or separation), illness, emotional or physical discomfort, uncomfortable sleeping environments (noise, light, heat or cold), and changes to the normal sleep schedule (e.g. due to travel). Acute insomnia often heals itself without any treatment with the passage of time or the disappearance of the cause. On the other hand, chronic insomnia has many causes, which are often interwoven. Special diagnoses and medical or non-medical (cognitive and behavioural) treatments are needed to cure it (National Sleep Foundation 2019).

Effects of chronic insomnia

Chronic insomnia increases the risk of somatic and psychiatric disorders, poor occupational performance and work disability (Paunio, Tuisku and Korhonen 2015).

Institute of Medicine (2006) suggested that sleep deprivation, particularly chronic insomnia, can have a wide range of effects on the cardiovascular, endocrine, immune and nervous systems. O'Connell (2017) provided a list of diseases that are caused by insomnia, namely: weak immune system, asthma attacks, seizures, inflammation, obesity, diabetes, high blood pressure, heart diseases and stroke. Khanijow et al. (2015) related sleep dysfunction with gastrointestinal diseases and reported strong relationships between sleep and diseases such as gastroesophageal reflux, peptic ulcer, irritable bowel syndrome, functional dyspepsia, inflammatory bowel, colorectal cancer and liver disease. Active Health (2019) alerted that chronic insomnia reduces life expectancy; the risk of early mortality is 97% higher in those who suffer from chronic insomnia.

The link between chronic insomnia and psychiatric disorders have been well-established in the epidemiological discipline. Baglioni et al. (2011) concluded in a meta-analysis of existing evidence that insomnia doubles the risk of developing depression in the subsequent years. Paunio et al. (2009) revealed a causal relationship between poor sleep quality and life dissatisfaction, mediated by neurophysiological effects on the brain, the emotions and depressed mood. Moreover, Paunio, Tuisku and Korhonen (2015) claimed that sleep disturbances lead to sensitivity symptoms, functional pains and fatigue. They further claimed that chronic work stress combined with chronic insomnia lead to burnout. O'Connell (2017) posited that insomnia increases the risk of depression, anxiety, confusion and frustration.

Insomnia impairs daily functioning and work performance. Salminen et al. (2010) claimed that insomnia impedes cognitive and social performance at work through tiredness, reduced attention and alertness, slowed response, and impaired memory and learning. They also increase the vulnerability to work injuries and errors in judgements (Paunio, Tuisku and Korhonen 2015). Balkin et al. (2008) reinforced that employees with sleep deprivation experience a decline in the quality of life and work productivity along with increased rates of accidents and errors at work. Léger et al. (2002) suggested that insomnia increases absenteeism from work. Lallukka et al. (2014) concurred that insomnia doubled sick leave days. This could be due to the combined psychosomatic consequences of insomnia. These collectively lead to an imbalance between work demand and actual performance, eventually leading to reduced achievements, lower job satisfaction and adverse career progression (Scott and Judge 2006).

Causes of chronic insomnia

Riba (1993) classified causes of chronic insomnia into four categories, namely: medical conditions, psychiatric conditions, medications and stimulants, and habits/lifestyle.

Chronic insomnia can be caused by pains and discomfort resulting from long-term medical conditions. To mention a few conditions: asthma, sinus allergies, acid reflux, hyperthyroidism, diabetes, congestive heart failure, arthritis, lower back pain, fibromyalgia, Parkinson's disease, restless leg syndrome, menopause and cancer (Santos-Longhurst 2018; National Sleep Foundation 2019).

Chronic insomnia can also be caused by psychiatric conditions such as chronic stress, anxiety, depression, bipolar disorder, obsessive compulsive disorder, hypomania, anorexia nervosa, schizophrenia, alcoholism and drug addiction (Riba 1993; Santos-Longhurst 2018). Paunio, Tuisku and Korhonen (2015) claimed that psychiatric conditions and insomnia have a bi-directional relationship and can become a vicious cycle.

In some people, the intake of certain regular medications and stimulants may cause chronic insomnia. Examples of such medications include thyroid hormones, anorexigenics, antidepressants, sympathomimetics, diuretics, beta-blockers, corticosteroids, reserpine and chemotherapy drugs (Riba 1993).

Certain lifestyles and habits can trigger insomnia. These are: frequent daytime napping, late physically stimulating activities (exercise), late intellectually stimulating activities (work at home in evenings), the light from computers or similar screens keeps the brain alert even after one goes to sleep, irregular sleeping hours and patterns, alcohol or tobacco use, and/or excessive caffeine intake (National Sleep Foundation 2019; Riba 1993).

In summary, chronic insomnia can be caused by a single or a combination of conditions in an individual. Moreover, often complex interplays are formed among medical conditions, psychiatric conditions and insomnia.

Work-related risk factors for chronic insomnia

The preceding section outlined the general causes of chronic insomnia. Work conditions and occupational settings can also lead to chronic insomnia. Åkerstedt et al. (2002) argued that work stress is the prime cause of persistent insomnia.

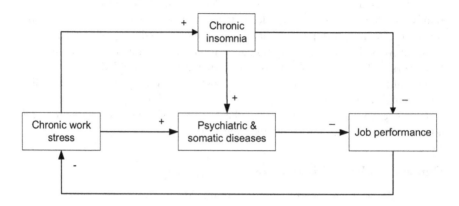

Figure 3.1 Work stress induced chronic insomnia

Source: Modified from Paunio, Tuisku and Korhonen 2015; and Pereira and Elfering 2014

Figure 3.1 depicts an overarching model, connecting work stress, insomnia, psychiatric and somatic diseases, and job performance, which was augmented from Paunio, Tuisku and Korhonen (2015) and Pereira and Elfering (2014). The model postulates a dynamic causal loop and a vicious cycle. On one hand, chronic work stress can directly cause psychiatric and somatic diseases. On the other hand, chronic work stress can trigger chronic insomnia, which in turn can cause and/or exacerbate psychiatric and somatic diseases, and fatigue. Subsequently, insomnia directly and through the psychiatric and somatic diseases pathway leads to reduced job performance, adding further work stressors such as diminished support from colleagues and the supervisor and/or job insecurity (Van Laethem et al. 2015; Kompier, Taris and van Veldhoven 2012). Evidence for the causal connections between work stressors and insomnia was elicited from occupational medicine literature and detailed in the ensuing section.

Healthy sleep is one of the most essential recovery mechanisms of the human body and the mind, after a busy workday. There is growing evidence that chronic work stress contributes to disturbed sleep quality, particularly chronic insomnia, and thereby causes incomplete/impaired recovery, which subsequently leads to diminished psychiatric and somatic health in the long run (Pereira and Elfering 2014; Lallukka, Rahkonen and Lahelma 2011; Åkerstedt, Nilsson and Kecklund 2009; Geurts and Sonnentag 2006). Researchers discovered many psychosocial stressors and work conditions that have resulted in chronic insomnia in the working population around the world:

- Pereira and Elfering (2014) empirically proved that social stressors at work are positively related to fragmented sleep (i.e. waking up repeatedly throughout the night), which mediated psychosomatic health complaints. They defined social stressors at work as workplace characteristics such as conflicts with colleagues, blaming culture, reduced tolerance for errors and deliberate unpleasant work assignments.

- Åkerstedt et al. (2002) claimed that overtime work/long working week and hectic work, interpreted as high work demand with low decision latitude, predicts sleep disturbances and fatigue. Similarly, Salo et al. (2014) and Linton et al. (2015) noted an increased prevalence of sleep disturbances among employees who experienced low control over working hours, high work demands, job strain, effort–reward imbalance and bullying. Ota et al. (2009) listed two additional factors such as low support and over commitment at work and Van Laethem et al. (2013) added job insecurity.

- Shift work is a well-established cause of sleep disorders in many research studies; the disturbance of the circadian rhythm, triggered by shift work, is regarded as the key mechanism for sleep disorders (Åkerstedt et al. 2002; Ribet and Derriennic 1999; Härmä et al. 1998). Moreover, shift workers have reported more job stress than daytime workers (Tenkanen et al. 1997). Conversely, Kalimo et al. (2000) concluded that the association between job stressors and sleep disorders (sleep deprivation and insomnia) was greater in daytime workers than shift workers. Nonetheless, they found the highest prevalence of insomnia and daytime fatigue among people who reported high demand and low control at work.

- Berset et al. (2011) argued that time pressure and effort–reward imbalance at work cause rumination, which in turn leads to impaired sleep. Knudsen, Ducharme and Roman (2007) posited that workload, role conflict, job autonomy and repetitive tasks were associated with poor sleep quality but out of the four variables, workload predicted poor sleep more strongly.

Existing literature discusses only selected psychosocial factors/work characteristics. Out of the discussed factors, job demands, job control and shift work were found to have a strong association with insomnia whilst the rest have a moderate association. However, recent job stress studies and well-known job stress instruments/inventories identity over 20 important stressors that have strong associations with job stress. Hence, further studies are required to investigate the degree of influence of all important stressors at work. Moreover, the presence and impact of stressors vary across industry sectors. For example, shift work has been highlighted in many studies of insomnia among nurses. The construction industry is unique, and therefore it is possible that there could be specific stressors and circumstances that challenge construction professionals. This is yet to be explored.

Confounders

Apart from the work-related factors discussed already, literature also suggests confounders that interfere with the association between work stress and sleep disorders. Åkerstedt et al. (2002) claimed that sleep disorders due to work-related factors are more prevalent among women and higher age groups (aged above 49 years). Existing long-term illness was found to be a strong confounder. Tenkanen et al. (1997) discovered confounding effects of age, smoking, alcohol and sedentary nature on the association between work stress and insomnia. However, Kalimo et al. (2000) refuted that lifestyle factors such as smoking, alcohol and sedentary behaviour as well as age were not significant confounders of the effects. Ota et al. (2009) argued that the occupational position or type, particularly managerial positions, were significantly related to persistent insomnia. Hence, it is important to examine the confounding factors related to construction professionals and chronic insomnia.

Research method

The preceding sections provided a literature background for chronic insomnia, work-related causes and consequences from a broader perspective. The remainder of the chapter investigates these empirically in the context of the Australian construction industry by traversing through the following research questions:

- What is the prevalence of work stress induced insomnia among construction professionals?
- What are the most significant job stressors causing insomnia?
- How do individual characteristics influence work stress induced insomnia?
- To what degree does work stress induced insomnia affect job outcomes?
- How do individual stress coping styles affect insomnia?
- How does work stress induced insomnia impact on physical and mental ill-health?

Data

The dataset required for this research was extracted from the complete data collected from the Australian construction industry using an online questionnaire survey. The details of the survey, its administration and respondents were discussed in Chapter 1 in the 'research methodology' section, and therefore are not repeated in this chapter, but the data related to the chapter are summarised in Table 3.2. A copy of the complete survey instrument can be found in the Appendix.

The survey was responded by 310 participants, but only 247 responses were complete and could be used for analysis. This was above the minimum required sample size of 241 for a survey that collects responses on a 4-point Likert scale, as per Park and Jung (2009). Refer to Table 1.3 in Chapter 1 for socio-demographic details of the survey respondents. Except for the socio-demographic details of the respondents, responses to most other questions were collected on 4-point textural Likert scales. The textual Likert scales used in the survey were coded numerically in the following manner to standardise and facilitate quantitative analyses:

- Scale 1: never = 0, sometimes = 1, often = 2, always = 3
- Scale 2: not satisfied = 0, somewhat satisfied = 1, satisfied = 2, very satisfied = 3
- Scale 3: never = 0, once or twice = 1, monthly = 2, weekly = 3
- Scale 4: not at all = 0, several days = 1, more than half the days = 2, nearly every day = 3

Table 3.2 Data related to work stress induced insomnia

Section	Response options

Respondent's background
1. Gender (male, female or other)
2. Age (≤20, 21–30, 31–40, 41–50, 51–60 or >60)
3. Marital status (married/de-facto, single or divorced/separated/widowed)
4. Organisation type (property development, PM, architecture, engineering, QS, builder, subcontractor, FM or other)
5. Organisation size (measured by # of full-time employees) (≤4, 5–19, 20–199 or ≥200)
6. Job title (text responses were received but categorised as junior professional, mid-career professional, senior professional or executive)
7. Experience (<1 year, 1–5 years, 6–10 years or >10 years)
8. Nature of employment (permanent, fixed-term contract or casual)
9. Hours worked weekly (<20, 20–30, 30–40, 40–50 or >50)
10. Workplace environment (site or office)
11. Income (<$40k, $40–60k, $60–80k, $80–100k, $100–120k, $120–150k or >$150k)

Job stressors

In the past 6 months at work how often did you experience:

Measured using the scale of:
- Never
- Sometimes
- Often
- Always

1. Poor/dangerous work environment
2. Excessive workload
3. Unpredictable work hours
4. Time pressure
5. Job autonomy
6. Job appropriateness
7. Flexibility
8. Supportive feedback
9. Line manager support
10. Co-worker support
11. Harassment
12. Bullying
13. Discrimination
14. Role ambiguity
15. Adequate job resources
16. Staff consultation
17. Sufficient remuneration
18. Reward
19. Job security
20. Career prospect

Work–private life interplay

In the past 6 months how often did you experience:

Measured using the scale of:
- Never
- Sometimes
- Often
- Always

1. Lack of energy for private life
2. Lack of time for private life
3. Family complained about too much work
4. Other personal life stressors

Chronic job stress

In the past 4 weeks how often did you experience:

Measured using the scale of:
- Never
- Sometimes
- Often
- Always

1. Poor sleep
2. Restlessness
3. Irritability
4. Tensed
5. Nervousness

(continued)

Table 3.2 Cont.

Section	Response options
Sleep problems/Insomnia	
A) In the past 6 months how often were you bothered by/treated for insomnia?	Measured using the scale of: • Never • Once or twice • Monthly • Weekly
B) Do you believe that your job is the primary cause?	Dichotomous response –Yes / No
Stress coping methods	
In the past 4 weeks how often did you engage in the following stress coping methods: 1. Problem-solving 2. Positive reappraisal 3. Seeking support 4. Relaxation 5. Physical activity 6. Leisure and humour 7. Eating balanced diet 8. Adequate sleep 9. Isolation 10. Alcohol/drug use 11. Smoking 12. Emotional eating 13. Criticise/blame others 14. Compulsive spending 15. Denial/ignoring as if nothing happened 16. Releasing tension	Measured using the scale of: • Not at all • Several days • More than half the days • Nearly every day
Physical and mental health effects	
A) In the past 6 months how often were you bothered by/treated for: 1. High blood pressure 2. High cholesterol 3. High blood sugar level 4. Angina 5. Heart muscle weakening 6. Heart attack 7. Stroke 8. Diabetes 9. Weight gain/obesity 10. Gastrointestinal disorders 11. Asthma 12. Bronchitis 13. Pneumonia 14. Eczema 15. Chronic headache/migraine 16. Back, neck or shoulder pain 17. Arthritis 18. Blurred eye vision 19. Slow healing 20. Sexual dysfunction 21. Reproductive system disorder	Measured using the scale of: • Never • Once or twice • Monthly • Weekly

Table 3.2 Cont.

Section	Response options
22. Burnout	
23. Anxiety	
24. Depression	
B) Do you believe that your job is the primary cause? (this was asked for each heath problem above)	Dichotomous response –Yes / No
Job outcomes	
In the past 6 months how would you rate your:	Measured using a scale of 1 (low) to
1. Job satisfaction	10 (high)
2. Job performance	

Data analysis techniques

Several analysis techniques were used to answer the research questions as follows:

- Analysis of measures of central tendency and one sample t-test were conducted to assess the prevalence of insomnia among construction professionals in general.
- Factorial ANOVA technique was deployed to investigate the influence of socio-demographic factors on insomnia experiences.
- Cluster analysis was undertaken to investigate the relationship of insomnia with job stressors, work stress, work–life conflict, stress coping, mental disorders and job outcomes. Cluster analysis is an analytics technique that helps grouping of data/responses based on their characteristics. Subsequently it enables the identification of most significant data/response characteristics that are pertinent to an outcome. Clustering analysis is a promising method for identifying and describing groups of individual cases, considering multiple dimensions/variables of interest simultaneously (Doron et al. 2014). It provides an advantage over traditional statistical techniques in delineating naturally occurring groups within data (Wijndaele et al. 2007; Hillhouse and Adler 1997).
- Associations between insomnia and physical health issues were explored using the Pearson bi-variate correlation technique.

Construction professionals and work-related chronic insomnia

This section expounds the findings of the analyses under relevant subheadings and discusses these alongside previous research findings.

Prevalence of chronic insomnia among construction professionals

Descriptive statistical analyses were conducted to understand insomnia prevalence and its severity spread among construction industry professionals who responded to the survey. Participants' responses to the following questions were analysed:

A) In the past 6 months how often were you bothered by/treated for insomnia?
    • Never
    • Once or twice
    • Monthly
    • Weekly

B) Do you believe that your job stress may have caused this illness?
    • No
    • Yes

Figure 3.2 illustrates the results. Forty percent of respondents indicated that they suffer from insomnia and it is induced by work stress. The severity level was assessed based on the frequency of treatment received. Figure 3.2(a) suggests that 15% of the respondents (around 38% of the sufferers) receive treatment as frequently as weekly and around 9% of the respondents (22% of the sufferers) are treated at least once a month. The remaining 16% (40% of the sufferers) received treatments a few times in the past 6 months.

The overall prevalence and severity levels were combinedly calculated using the mean of the responses received and the numerical coding used for the textual responses. Then, one sample t-test was conducted to check whether the inferred population mean is significantly different from that of the sample that responded to the survey. The results are shown in Figure 3.3. The p-value of .879, which is greater than the threshold p-value of .05, suggests that the insomnia level of the population of professionals is not significantly different from that of the sample surveyed. It can therefore be concluded that 40% of construction industry professionals in Australia suffer from work-related insomnia and more than one-third of them obtain treatment as frequently as weekly and about another quarter of them receive treatment monthly.

There have been several studies globally to assess the prevalence of insomnia in the adult population, which found varying proportions of people who suffer from it in different regions of the world. For instance, studies conducted in Canada found that around 20% of the general adult population suffer from insomnia (Sutton, Moldofsky and Badley 2001). This figure was inconsistent with later reports from other western countries such as Britain (Groeger, Zijlstra and Dijk 2004), Finland (Kronholm et al. 2006) and the United States (Stranges et al. 2008). Cross-continent studies of Stranges et al. (2012), which was conducted in countries in Africa (Ghana, Tanzania, South Africa and Kenya) and Asia (India, Bangladesh, Vietnam and Indonesia), revealed a range from 4% to 40%. Roth (2007) reconciled these varying statistics that approximately 30% of a variety of

(a) Prevalence and severity spread

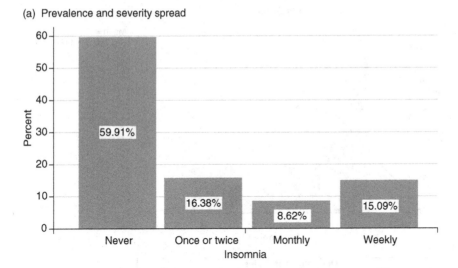

(b) Work induced or not

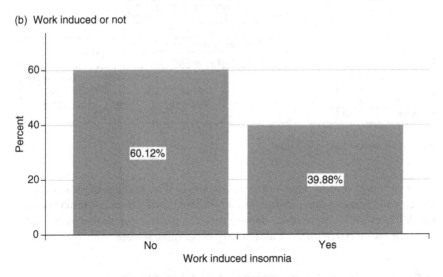

Figure 3.2 Prevalence of work induced insomnia

adult samples drawn from different countries report one or more of the symptoms of insomnia. A recent study conducted within the Australian general population discovered that the prevalence of self-reported doctor-diagnosed insomnia varied little across age groups (25 to 34 years – 7.4%; 65 to 74 years – 6.8%), although it was higher in 18 to 24 years (12.5%) (Reynolds et al. 2019). In the context of the construction industry, many studies around the world have reported that construction professionals generally experience sleep problems, but the level of

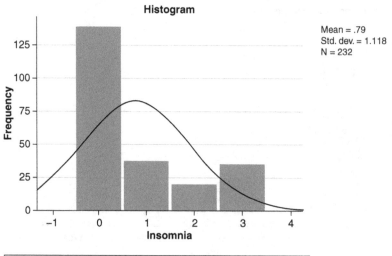

Histogram

Mean = .79
Std. dev. = 1.118
N = 232

One-sample statistics				
	N	Mean	Std. deviation	Std. error mean
Insomnia	232	.79	1.118	.073

One-sample test						
	Test value = 0.8					
					95% Confidence interval of the difference	
				Mean		
	t	df	Sig. (2-tailed)	difference	Lower	Upper
Insomnia	−.153	231	.879	−.011	−.16	.13

Figure 3.3 One sample t-test results

prevalence and severity have not been identified. The findings of this study fill this gap and suggests that construction professionals suffer from insomnia at a rate much higher (40%) (more than double) than the general population in Australia and other western countries. This is a very concerning statistic.

Influence of socio-demographic factors on insomnia

The influences of socio-demographic factors such as gender, age, organisation type and organisation size on insomnia experiences were tested using Factorial ANOVA. As for gender and age, answers for the following questions were sought:

- Do the age and gender have an impact on insomnia experiences?
- Is there an interaction between age and gender on insomnia experiences?

Table 3.3 presents the factorial ANOVA test results for age and gender influences on insomnia. The p-values yielded for both gender and age are below the threshold

Table 3.3 Factorial ANOVA results for age and gender

Tests of between-subjects effects

Dependent variable: insomnia

Source	Type III sum of squares	df	Mean square	F	Sig.
Corrected model	40.340[a]	14	2.881	2.518	.002
Intercept	25.813	1	25.813	22.558	.000
Gender	10.015	2	5.008	4.376	.014
Age	25.131	6	4.188	3.660	.002
Gender x Age	9.591	6	1.598	1.397	.217
Error	248.311	217	1.144		
Total	433.000	232			
Corrected total	288.651	231			

a. R Squared = .140 (Adjusted R Squared = .084)

value of .05, suggesting that there are significant differences in insomnia experience across different age groups and genders. However, the p-value for the interaction between age and gender to influence insomnia (p-value = .217) is greater than the threshold p-value of .05. There is no significant influence by their interaction. This is further reinforced by the plot shown in Figure 3.4. Insomnia experience is increased with age and it is more prevalent and severe among female professionals.

In studying insomnia among the Australian general population, Reynolds et al. (2019) reported that doctor-diagnosed insomnia was more common in females (8.6%) than males (6.2%). Similarly, Stranges et al. (2012) found a consistent pattern of higher prevalence of sleep problems in women and older groups in their studies of Asian and African countries. Same patterns were observed in Canada by Morin et al. (2011) that insomnia was strongly associated with females, older age and poorer self-rated physical and mental health. However, in the construct industry of South Africa, Bowen et al. (2018) claimed that less experienced/junior female professionals showed higher insomnia symptoms. The present study's findings concur with the patterns among the general population across many countries, including Australia, but contradicts with Bowen et al. (2018) in one facet about construction professionals. That is, in Australia insomnia is more prevalent among older/senior female professionals. This could possibly be linked to increasing responsibilities with age/seniority at both work and home/family.

Table 3.4 presents the factorial ANOVA results for testing the effects of organisation size and workplace type on insomnia experience. The p-value for organisation size (.047) is smaller than .05, suggesting that the size of the organisation has a significant influence on insomnia experience. On the contrary, workplace type, whether office or site based, is not significant. As further explained by Figure 3.5, professionals in micro organisations experienced insomnia more often followed

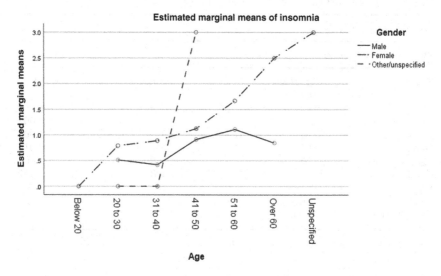

Figure 3.4 Effects of age and gender on insomnia

Table 3.4 Factorial ANOVA results for organisation size and workplace type

Tests of between-subjects effects

Dependent variable: insomnia

Source	Type III sum of squares	df	Mean square	F	Sig.
Corrected model	13.489[a]	7	1.927	1.590	.139
Intercept	85.640	1	85.640	70.666	.000
Organisation size	9.801	3	3.267	2.696	.047
Workplace	.797	1	.797	.657	.418
Organisation size x Workplace	.657	3	.219	.181	.910
Error	270.252	223	1.212		
Total	424.000	231			
Corrected total	283.740	230			

a. R Squared = .048 (Adjusted R Squared = .018)

by medium sized organisations. In the construction industry many micro sized organisations are run by a single person as sole trader or a few who take care of all aspects of the business. This may contribute to increased stress and thereby insomnia.

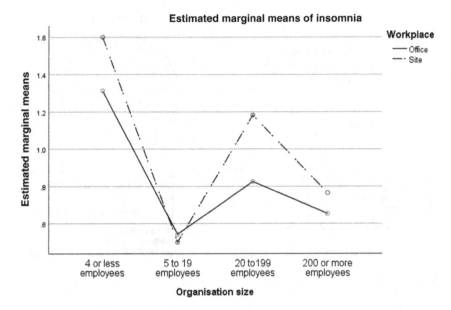

Figure 3.5 Effects of organisation size and workplace on insomnia

Chronic insomnia cluster analysis

To identify and classify naturally occurring patterns of relationships of insomnia with job stressors, stress, stress coping styles, mental disorders and job performance, clustering was conducted using IBM SPSS 26.0. Three clustering techniques are available in IBM SPSS, namely K-means clustering, hierarchical clustering and TwoStep clustering. K-means clustering is a non-hierarchical clustering technique which can be used to perform clustering only based on continuous variables. Similarly, the hierarchical clustering technique processes only continuous variables. The TwoStep clustering is a combination of non-hierarchical and hierarchical techniques and it can process both categorical and continuous data for clustering. Hence, this study used the TwoStep clustering approach. Accordingly, the cluster analysis was conducted in two episodes, involving two successive steps as follows:

- TwoStep clustering technique was used to group the cases into n = k clusters by maximising between-cluster differences and minimising within-cluster variance in insomnia and other variables concerned.
- Statistical tests for the significance of cluster mean differences were applied to verify whether the clusters differed significantly for all variables included in the analysis.

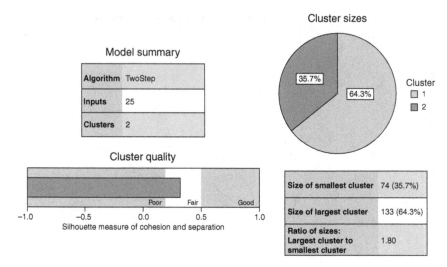

Figure 3.6 Clustering episode 1 summary

The first episode of cluster analysis was performed to investigate insomnia and its relationship with work stress, stressors, work–private life conflict and job outcomes. The analysis included: all the 20 stressors assessed in the survey, work stress, work–private life conflict, two indicators of job outcome such as job satisfaction and performance/productivity levels, and insomnia experience. The constructs such as work stress and work–private life conflict were represented by five and four indicators, respectively. Hence, the aggregated mean for these constructs were used. The analysis resulted in two clusters with a ratio of sizes with a value of 1.80, which is smaller than the preferred maximum threshold value of 2.00 (see Figure 3.6). Cluster 1 is almost double the size of cluster 2; cluster 1 is 64.3%; cluster 2 is 35.7%.

Table 3.5 presents the strength of the stressors and other insomnia causes across the clusters. It also shows the t-test results that investigated the significance of mean differences of the stressors and other insomnia causes across the clusters. The p-values yielded for all the variables are less than the significant value of .05, suggesting that the mean values of responses yielded for the variables across the clusters are significantly different and the two clusters represent two significantly different experiences of construction professionals. Cluster 2 appears to represent professionals who are significantly affected/suffer from work-related insomnia (mean = 1.49) and perceived work stress (mean = 1.84), with values more than double that of cluster 1 (mean values of .5 and .83 for insomnia and perceived work stress, respectively). Moreover, their level of job satisfaction is below average (mean value of 4.180 out of 10) and their job performance is average too (mean value of 5.81 out of 10).

Table 3.5 Results of clustering episode 1

	Cluster 1		Cluster 2		T-test results	
	Mean	S	Mean	S	t - stat.	Sig. (2 tailed)
Insomnia	.50	.901	1.49	1.263	−6.536	.000
Work stress	.8331	.515	1.835	.61964	−12.456	.000
Job outcome:						
How would you rate the level of satisfaction with your current job (1 = low; 10 = high)?	7.68	1.400	4.180	1.823	15.468	.000
How would you rate your overall job performance on the days you worked during the past 4 weeks?	7.95	1.381	5.81	2.162	8.692	.000
Stressors:						
I had to work in poor or dangerous physical work conditions	.14	.372	.58	.683	−5.982	.000
I had excessive workload	1.11	.659	2.11	.732	−10.006	.000
I had unpredictable work hours	1.14	.629	2.18	.690	−10.932	.000
I had excessive time pressure	.98	.798	1.47	.864	−4.095	.000
I had a choice/say in deciding how I do my work	2.09	.793	1.49	.832	5.161	.000
The work I performed was appropriate for my skills and abilities	2.47	.598	2.01	.712	4.953	.000
I had flexibility with my work time	2.25	.722	1.55	.724	6.621	.000
I was given supportive feedback on the work I did	2.06	.694	.96	.535	11.829	.000
I could rely on my line manager to help me out with a work problem	2.02	.917	1.03	.793	7.847	.000
If work got difficult, my colleagues helped me	2.14	.877	1.27	.849	6.879	.000
I was subject to harassment in the form of unkind/unwanted words or behaviour at work	2.08	.785	1.12	.661	8.850	.000
I was subject to bullying at work	1.95	.824	.99	.731	8.427	.000
I was subject to discrimination due to my gender, age or ethnic background	.10	.298	.86	.782	−10.087	.000
I was clear what my duties and responsibilities were	.08	.349	.70	.806	−7.678	.000
I had enough resources to do my work	.16	.405	.55	.724	−5.051	.000
I was consulted on matters/changes that affected my job	1.68	.932	1.07	.764	4.853	.000
My salary was sufficient for the work I had to do	1.95	.886	1.23	.803	5.829	.000
I had job security	2.42	.618	1.57	.980	7.673	.000
I received reward/appreciation for the efforts I put in	2.15	.723	1.19	.805	8.798	.000
I had career progress opportunities	1.95	.907	.960	.766	7.924	.000
Work–life conflict	.9981	.575	1.777	.63376	−9.000	.000

Observations of mean values yielded for stressors reveal that construction professionals who are represented by cluster 2 experienced the following stressors more often:

- excessive workload
- unpredictable work hours
- work–life conflict
- lack of support and feedback from co-workers and line managers
- lack of recognitions for efforts (effort–reward imbalance)
- job insecurity
- lack of career prospect.

These factors have contributed to insomnia and low job satisfaction and thereby reduced job performance. The predictor importance diagram shown in Figure 3.7 identifies harassment and discrimination also as important factors in creating these clusters. Whilst discrimination is relevant to cluster 2 at a lower degree (mean = .86), harassment has been experienced by professionals in cluster 1 more (mean values of 2.08 and 1.12 for cluster 1 and 2, respectively).

The second episode of clustering was performed to investigate insomnia and its relationship with stress coping style, mental disorders and job outcomes, which also resulted in two clusters with a ratio of sizes with a value of 1.70, which is smaller than the preferred maximum threshold value of 2.00 (see Figure 3.8). Akin to the previous clustering output, this episode produced similar size clusters (cluster 1: 37%; cluster 2: 63%).

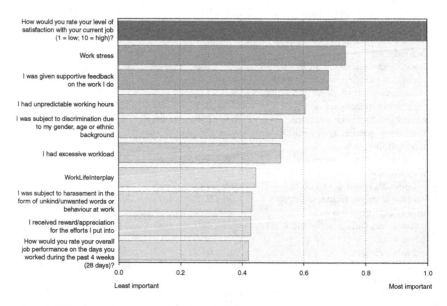

Figure 3.7 Predictor importance for clustering 1

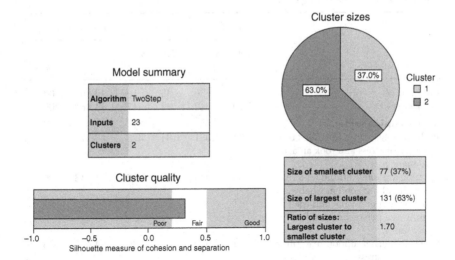

Figure 3.8 Clustering episode 2 summary

Table 3.6 reveals: (1) the mental disorders and job outcomes of suffering work stress related insomnia; and (2) the stress coping styles that are conducive to these outcomes. It also shows t-test results that investigated the significance of mean differences of insomnia, work stress, mental disorders, job outcomes and coping styles across the clusters. The p-values yielded suggest that the mean values of most indicators across the clusters are significantly different and the two clusters represent two significantly different experiences of construction professionals.

Cluster 1 represents construction professionals who are significantly affected by work stress induced insomnia (mean values of 1.79 and 1.70 for work stress and insomnia, respectively; the insomnia level is almost five times that of cluster 2) and mental disorders such as burnout (mean = 1.73; almost seven times that of cluster 2), anxiety (mean = 2.04; more than quadruple that of cluster 2) and depression (mean = 1.75; more than six times that of cluster 2). Moreover, their job satisfaction is below average (mean value of 4.74 out of 10) but their job performance is not significantly below cluster 2 (mean values of 6.23 and 7.78 for cluster 1 and 2, respectively). This suggests that despite high levels of perceived work stress, insomnia, mental disorders and job dissatisfaction, their productivity is not badly reduced, only a slight drop is discernible.

Comparisons of mean values of stress coping styles in the clusters suggest that professionals in cluster 1 apply adaptive coping methods to the similar level as professionals in cluster 2. However, they simultaneously resort to certain maladaptive coping styles substantially. Examples for such habits are consuming alcohol/drugs, emotional eating, sedentary behaviour, blaming others and denial/distancing. These affect their sleeping and relaxation abilities, contributing to

Table 3.6 Results of clustering episode 2

	Cluster 1		Cluster 2		T-test results	
	Mean	S	Mean	S	t-stat.	Sig. (2-tailed)
Insomnia	1.70	1.236	.35	.712	10.004	.000
Work stress	1.79	.642	.82	.517	11.962	.000
Stress coping style:						
Problem-solving (e.g. identified the source of stress and took an action to manage it)	1.34	1.021	.84	.875	3.722	.000
Keeping a positive attitude (I looked for something good in what was happening in my life and tried to grow as a person as a result of the situation)	1.56	1.032	1.40	1.073	1.013	.000
Seeking external support (e.g. talked about the stressful event with a supportive person/counsellor/ friend/colleague)	1.44	1.032	.86	.839	4.406	.000
Relaxation (e.g. engaged in meditation, breathing exercise, nature exposure and/or progressive muscle relaxation)	.78	.868	.61	.846	1.374	.171
Physical activity (engaged in team sports, exercise, yoga and/or swimming)	.90	.968	1.17	.978	−1.943	.053
Engaged in humour, fun and leisure activities (gardening, movie and/ or socialising)	1.21	.864	1.47	.880	−2.055	.041
Eating well-balanced meals	1.68	.910	1.77	.965	−.705	.482
Resting and sleeping enough	.87	.750	1.64	.953	−6.077	.000
Escape – isolating from others and making yourself busy with TV, reading, internet, etc.	1.71	1.037	1.29	.949	3.008	.003
Numbing – consuming alcohol or drugs to forget the stressful situation	1.39	1.090	.47	.705	7.357	.000
Smoking to get a relief from stress	.47	.940	.17	.543	2.916	.004
Emotional eating and drinking (eating comfort food and/or drinking coffee and other caffeine drinks to get relief from stress)	1.90	1.033	.77	.873	8.375	.000
Criticising or blaming others for the situation	1.55	1.020	.36	.569	10.772	.000
Compulsive spending – shopping and buying gifts for yourself to feel happy and forget stress	.75	.845	.31	.494	4.825	.000
Ignoring as if nothing happened/ trying to forget the whole thing (denial/distancing)	1.26	1.044	.47	.672	6.609	.000

Table 3.6 Cont.

	Cluster 1		Cluster 2		T-test results	
	Mean	*S*	*Mean*	*S*	*t-stat.*	*Sig. (2-tailed)*
Releasing tension by crying, yelling, throwing things, etc.	.74	.894	.18	.402	6.242	.000
Mental disorders:						
Burnout	1.73	1.084	.25	.501	13.353	.000
Anxiety	2.04	.952	.46	.671	13.999	.000
Depression	1.75	1.053	.27	.478	13.914	.000
Job outcome:						
How would you rate the level of satisfaction with your current job (1 = low; 10 = high)?	4.74	2.375	7.44	1.560	−9.895	.000
How would you rate your overall job performance on the days you worked during the past 4 weeks?	6.23	2.350	7.78	1.443	−5.877	.000

psychological outcomes such as burnout, anxiety and depression. This is confirmed by the predictor importance diagram depicted in Figure 3.9.

Bowen et al. (2018) have previously investigated insomnia among construction professionals in South Africa and found three strong predictors, namely psychological distress, job pressure and work–family conflict (in the descending order of prediction strength). Job pressure and work–family conflict exert both a direct influence on sleep problems and an indirect influence through psychological distress. This study confirms that psychological distress manifested as anxiety, depression, burnout and/or stress is the strongest determinant of chronic insomnia among construction professionals in Australia too. It also confirms that work pressure, represented by unpredictable work hours and excessive workload, and work–life conflict are also significant predictors of insomnia in Australia. Nevertheless, this study finds few more strong predictors of insomnia which were not discovered previously, which are job insecurity, lack of support, effort–reward imbalance, career stagnation, and harassment, bullying and discrimination.

Though rare in construction literature, repeated arguments are evident in occupational epidemiological literature about insomnia, psychiatric conditions and work performance:

- Existing literature argues that chronic work stress leads to chronic insomnia, which then contributes to the development of psychiatric conditions (Pereira and Elfering 2014; Lallukka, Rahkonen and Lahelma 2011). However, this study reveals the presence of a new factor in the causal relationship as well as a different order of events, i.e. chronic work stress, combined with the use of maladaptive coping methods, leads to psychiatric conditions that cause

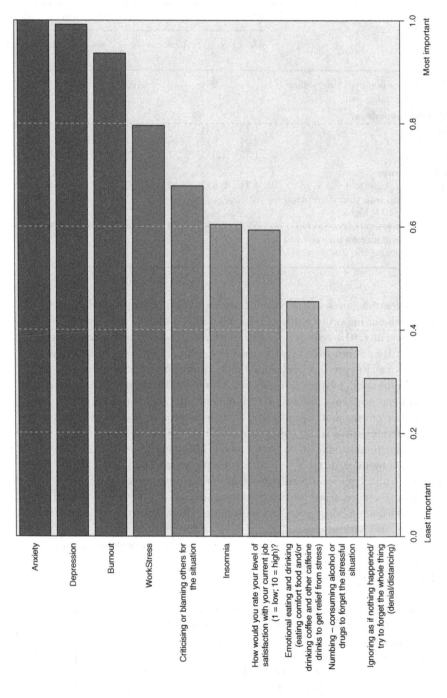

Figure 3.9 Predictor importance for clustering 2

chronic insomnia. When reconciled between the existing literature and the current findings, a bi-directional, vicious relationship can be deduced between insomnia and psychiatric conditions.

• Van Laethem et al. (2015), and Kompier, Taris and van Veldhoven (2012) argued that insomnia directly and through the psychiatric and somatic disease pathways leads to decreased job performance, which in turn adds more work stressors such as job insecurity. However, findings from this study revealed that construction professionals who experience work stress induced insomnia had lower job satisfaction, but their job productivity level was not considerably lower than others.

Association between insomnia and physical diseases among construction professionals

Table 3.7 shows the results of a correlation analysis between insomnia and other physical diseases among construction industry professionals. The correlation coefficient for a given association can range from −1.0 to +1.0 with the minus sign

Table 3.7 Associations between insomnia and diseases

Health problem	Insomnia	
	Correlation coefficient	*Sig. (2 tailed)*
Blurred eye vision	.552**	.000
Gastrointestinal disorders	.424**	.000
Weight gain/Obesity	.380**	.000
Arthritis	.380**	.000
Migraine or chronic headache	.361**	.000
Back, neck or shoulder pain	.344**	.000
High blood pressure	.336**	.000
Bronchitis	.285**	.000
Weakened immune system/slow healing	.268**	.000
Sexual dysfunction	.253**	.000
Reproductive system disorders	.238**	.000
High cholesterol	.232**	.000
Angina	.225**	.001
Heart attack	.210**	.001
Heart muscle weakening	.200**	.002
High blood sugar level	.177**	.007
Pneumonia	.168*	.011
Eczema	.161*	.014
Stroke	.157*	.017
Asthma	.115	.082
Diabetes type 2	.042	.530

** Correlation is significant at the .01 level (2-tailed).
* Correlation is significant at the .05 level (2-tailed).

(−) denoting a negative correlation and the plus sign (+) for a positive correlation between the concerned variables. The strength of the correlation is determined by the coefficient value. Nardi (2014) suggested that coefficients below .30 are considered weak, those between .30 to .70 are moderate and those above .70 are strong. Based on this guideline it can be deduced that insomnia and other physical diseases co-exist among construction industry professionals with some of the diseases having moderately strong associations while others have weak associations. Diseases with moderately strong associations, in the descending order, are blurred eye vision, gastrointestinal disorders, weight gain/obesity, arthritis, migraine or chronic headache, musculoskeletal pains and high blood pressure. Moreover, all the correlations are positive, meaning that with increased insomnia, the said disease condition also aggravates.

Existing epidemiological literature argues that chronic insomnia can cause a myriad of physical diseases such as: stroke, asthma attacks, seizures, weak immune system, sensitivity to pain, inflammation, obesity, diabetes, high blood pressure, heart diseases, gastroesophageal reflux, peptic ulcer, irritable bowel syndrome, functional dyspepsia, inflammatory bowel, colorectal cancer, liver disease, arthritis and visual impairment (Institute of Medicine 2006; O'Connell 2017; Khanijow et al. 2015; Seixas et al. 2014). This study confirms the associations between insomnia and most of the listed diseases with varying strengths of correlation. However, construction professionals are more vulnerable to insomnia induced diseases such as vision impairment, gastrointestinal disorders, weight gain/obesity, musculoskeletal and joint pains, and hypertension. Furthermore, it is noteworthy that construction professionals who suffer from insomnia may be vulnerable to rapid vision loss.

Cognitive behaviour therapy for treating insomnia

The preceding sections discussed the factors that cause insomnia among professionals in the Australian construction industry. Earlier sections discussed the importance of healthy sleep for good mental and physical health as well as performance. Hence, regardless of the work stressors encountered, construction professionals need to adopt strategies that can enable them to have adequate healthy sleep. Often individuals resort to sleeping medications to control insomnia, which may give immediate relief, but they may not be best in the long-term to treat insomnia. Cognitive behaviour therapy for insomnia (CBT-I) is instead recommended as an effective alternative as a long-term solution for insomnia, though it may take time and effort to make it work.

The cognitive part of CBT-I requires recognising and changing beliefs that affect his/her ability to sleep. It involves positive reappraisal of the circumstances and controlling or eliminating negative thoughts and worries that keep one awake. The behaviour part of CBT-I helps one develop good sleep habits and avoid behaviours that prevent one from sleeping well. The following behaviour modifications are recommended under CBT-I (Riba 1993, p17):

1. Go to bed only when you are actually sleepy but have a consistent time when you plan to go to sleep.
2. Do not use your bed for anything but sleep. No activities in bed like reading, watching TV, eating, talking on the phone, discussing problems or worrying in bed. Only exception to this is sexual relationship.
3. Set the alarm to get up at the same time every morning, regardless of how much sleep you had during the night or how tired you may be.
4. Do not nap during the day.
5. Do not drink alcohol within several hours before bedtime.
6. Do not smoke within several hours before bedtime.
7. Do not consume caffeine beverages or medications that contain caffeine within several hours before bedtime.
8. Exercise regularly in the later afternoon or early evening.
9. Allow yourself a transition period; during the hour before you go to bed, gradually decrease your activity level. Do things that are quiet and relaxing and avoid physically or mentally stimulating activities (e.g. late exercise, computer use).
10. Develop a routine before going to bed to make you feel comfortable, safe and secure; for example – personal hygiene, checking lights, locking doors.
11. Make sure no excessive light or noise will disturb your sleep and that your room is at a comfortable temperature.
12. Going to bed hungry or after a large meal can inhibit sleep. However, if you feel hungry have a light snack or a glass of warm milk.

Conclusion

The present study contributes new knowledge about chronic insomnia as a serious work health and safety consideration, which has long been underexplored in construction literature. The study reveals the following key insights, which are diagrammatically explained in Figure 3.10:

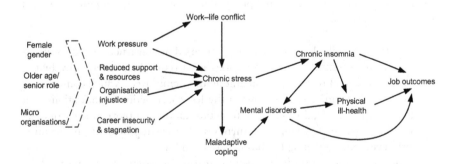

Figure 3.10 Consolidation of research findings

- Around 40% of professionals in the Australian construction industry suffer from moderate to severe chronic insomnia – a proportion that is more than double the rate in the Australian general population.
- Chronic insomnia is more prevalent among senior female professionals than their counterpart in the Australian construction industry.
- Professionals attached to micro sized organisations (i.e. organisations with four or less employees) suffer from more severe insomnia than those professionals attached to large organisations in Australia. This is likely due to the trend in the Australian construction industry that most micro organisations are sole traders or partnerships between few people. They have the responsibility for managing all affairs of the business and for ensuring the continuity of the business.
- The prevalence of five key phenomena in the local industry acts as root determinants of the higher rate of chronic insomnia, which are: excessive work pressure, reduced support and resources, organisational injustice, career insecurity and stagnation, and work–life conflict. These factors lead to chronic work stress that mediates chronic insomnia.
- Professionals who choose certain maladaptive coping techniques to manage work stress become increasingly vulnerable to psychiatric conditions such as anxiety, burnout and depression. Among the rampant maladaptive stress coping methods in the Australian construction industry are alcohol or drug use, emotional eating, sedentary behaviour, blaming and denial/distancing.
- Psychiatric conditions further increase the vulnerability to chronic insomnia, which in turn worsens psychiatric conditions, resulting in a vicious cycle.
- Chronic insomnia has caused a moderate reduction in the productivity level but a higher job dissatisfaction level among construction professionals in Australia.
- Construction professionals who suffer from chronic insomnia are more likely to contract physical diseases such as rapid vision loss, gastrointestinal disorders, obesity, musculoskeletal and joint pains, and hypertension.

The findings and the analytics methods applied in the study have valuable practical implications for individual professionals, construction organisations and healthcare specialists.

- The study identified psychosocial risk factors that construction organisations should aim to eliminate from their workplaces to curtail the onset of psychiatric conditions and chronic insomnia among their employees, which compromise their job performance. It is noteworthy for construction organisations that these risk factors lead to job dissatisfaction among employees, subsequently resulting in increased employee turnover, and re-employment and training costs, eventually affecting the business bottom line.
- Female construction professionals in construction organisations, particularly those at senior levels and/or with growing families, may require more flexible

arrangements than male professionals and those female professionals who have no carer responsibilities. Construction organisations and the industry in general could consider having modified employment terms for female professionals with carer responsibilities. This will not only help address the problem of work stress induced insomnia but also retain and grow female representation in the construction industry. It is acknowledged that some other sectors have more flexible and modified work arrangements for the said cohort of employees, but the construction industry is lagging. There are lessons and insights that the construction industry could draw from other similar sectors in the economy.

- Small scale organisations represent a significant portion of the local construction industry and their business sustainability is critical to the industry and the overall economy. However, the proprietors of those organisations are vulnerable to increased stress, chronic insomnia, psychiatric conditions and chronic physical diseases. This can eventually cause instability of small organisations and health and mental sufferings for the proprietors and their families. The state and local governments could devise a support system for small construction businesses to enable them to manage their businesses and life affairs smoothly regardless of market cycles. The support system could cover aspects related to economic/financial management through industry mentoring and training to subsidies and incentives.

- Individual professionals who are exposed to excessive work stress should improve their ability to exercise mindfulness and resilience to negative stress coping methods and increase regular physical and leisure activities as a priority in life. It is important to internalise that adopting shortcut measures to cope with stress is physically and psychologically dangerous, which can damage them and their families extensively. Seeking support from external cognitive behaviour consultants/therapists and faithfully adopting their guidelines is highly advised if one faces difficulty sleeping due to work problems.

- Healthcare and mental health specialists who treat and/or counsel construction professionals for chronic insomnia could utilise the findings of this study to perform a thorough analysis of risk factors for the condition. It also informs healthcare specialists who treat construction professionals of possible risk factors insomnia and physical disease complaints such as impaired eyesight, gastrointestinal disorders, obesity, musculoskeletal and joint pains, and hypertension.

- Cluster analysis techniques offer the potential for construction organisations to identify employees at high risk of insomnia, psychiatric conditions and related physical diseases, based on their stress coping styles and demographic factors. This can enable pro-active interventions to be developed and targeted appropriately in a cost-effective manner rather than using a general, one-size-fits-all approach. Similarly, the approach can help healthcare specialists in identifying construction professionals who are vulnerable to imminent mental disorders and chronic diseases.

References

Active Health. (2019). How does insomnia affect your life? Retrieved 12 December, 2019, from www.myactivesg.com/active-health/read/2019/2/how-does-insomnia-affect-your-life.

Åkerstedt, T. and Nilsson, P.M. (2003). Sleep as restitution: an introduction. *Journal of Internal Medicine, 254*(1), 6–12.

Åkerstedt, T., Fredlund, P., Gillberg, M. and Jansson, B. (2002). Workload and work hours in relation to disturbed sleep and fatigue in a large representative sample. *Journal of Psychosomatic Research, 53*(1), 585–588.

Åkerstedt, T., Nilsson, P.M. and Kecklund, G. (2009). Sleep and recovery. In S. Sonnentag, P.L. Perrewé and D.C. Ganster (Eds.), *Current Perspectives on Job-Stress Recovery: Research in Occupational Stress and Wellbeing* (Vol. 7, pp205–247). Bingley, UK: Emerald Group Publishing Limited.

American Psychiatric Association. (2019). What are sleep disorders? Retrieved 13 December, 2019, from www.psychiatry.org/patients-families/sleep-disorders/what-are-sleep-disorders.

Baglioni, C., Battagliese, G., Feige, B., Spiegelhalder, K., Nissen, C., Voderholzer, U., Lombardo, C. and Riemann, D. (2011). Insomnia as a predictor of depression: a meta-analytic evaluation of longitudinal epidemiological studies. *Journal of Affective Disorders, 135*(1–3), 10–19.

Balkin, T.J., Rupp, T., Picchioni, D. and Wesensten, N.J. (2008). Sleep loss and sleepiness: current issues. *Chest, 134*(3), 653–660.

Berset, M., Elfering, A., Luthi, S. and Semmer, N.K. (2011). Work stressors and impaired sleep: rumination as a mediator. *Stress and Health, 27*(2), e71–e82.

Bowen, P., Govender, R., Edwards, P. and Cattell, K. (2018). Work-related contact, work-family conflict, psychological distress and sleep problems experienced by construction professionals: an integrated explanatory model. *Construction Management and Economics, 36*(3), 153–174.

Doron, J., Trouillet, R., Maneveau, A., Neveu, D. and Ninot, G. (2014). Coping profiles, perceived stress and health-related behaviors: a cluster analysis approach. *Health Promotion International, 30*(1), 88–100.

Geurts, S.A.E. and Sonnentag, S. (2006). Recovery as an explanatory mechanism in the relation between acute stress reactions and chronic health impairment. *Scandinavian Journal of Work, Environment & Health, 32*(6), 482–492.

Groeger, J.A., Zijlstra, F.R. and Dijk, D.J. (2004). Sleep quantity, sleep difficulties and their perceived consequences in a representative sample of some 2000 British adults. *J Sleep Res, 13*, 359–371.

Härmä, M. (2013). Psychological work characteristics and sleep – a well-known but poorly understood association. *Scandinavian Journal of Work, Environment and Health, 39*(6), 531–533.

Härmä, M., Tenkanen, L., Sjöblom, T., Alikoski, T. and Heinsalmi, P. (1998). Combined effects of shift work and life-style on the prevalence of insomnia, sleep deprivation and daytime sleepiness. *Scandinavian Journal of Work, Environment and Health, 24*(4), 300–307.

Hillhouse, J.J. and Adler, C.M. (1997). Investigating stress effect patterns in hospital staff nurses: results of a cluster analysis. *Social Science and Medicine, 45*(12), 1781–1788.

Hossain, J.L. and Shapiro, C.M. (2002). The prevalence, cost implications, and management of sleep disorders: an overview. *Sleep Breath, 6*, 85–102.

Institute of Medicine. (2006). *Sleep Disorders and Sleep Deprivations: An Unmet Public Health Problem.* Washington, DC: The National Academies Press.

Kalimo, R., Tetikanen, L., Härmä, M., Poppius, E. and Heinsalmi, P. (2000). Job stress and sleep disorders: findings from the Helsinki heart study. *Stress Medicine, 16*(2), 65–75.

Khanijow, V., Prakash, P., Emsellem, H.A., Borum, M.L. and Doman, D.B. (2015). Sleep dysfunction and gastrointestinal diseases. *Gastroenterology & Hepatology, 11*(12), 817–825.

Knudsen, H.K., Ducharme, L.J. and Roman, P.M. (2007). Job stress and poor sleep quality: data from an American sample of full-time workers. *Social Science & Medicine, 64*(10), 1997–2007.

Kompier, M.A., Taris, T.W. and van Veldhoven, M. (2012). Tossing and turning: Insomnia in relation to occupational stress, rumination, fatigue, and well-being. *Scandinavian Journal of Work, Environment and Health, 38*(3), 238–246. http://dx.doi.org/10.5271/sjweh.3263.

Kronholm, E., Harma, M., Hublin, C., Aro, A.R. and Partonen, T. (2006). Self-reported sleep duration in Finnish general population. *Journal of Sleep Research, 15*(3), 276–290.

Lallukka, T., Kaikkonen, R., Härkänen, T., Kronholm, E., Partonen, T., Rahkonen, O. and Koskinen, S. (2014). Sleep and sickness absence: a nationally representative register-based follow-up study. *Sleep, 37*(9), 1413–1425.

Lallukka, T., Rahkonen, O. and Lahelma, E. (2011). Workplace bullying and subsequent sleep problems—the Helsinki Health Study. *Scandinavian Journal of Work, Environment & Health, 37*(3), 204–212.

Léger, D., Guilleminault, C., Bader, G., Lévy, E. and Paillard, M. (2002). Medical and socio-professional impact of insomnia. *Sleep, 25*(6), 625–629.

Linton, S.J., Kecklund, G., Franklin, K.A., Leissner, L.C., Sivertsen, B., Lindberg, E., Svensson, A.C., Hansson, S.O., Sundin, Ö., Hetta, J., Björkelund, C. and Hall, C. (2015). The effect of the work environment on future sleep disturbances: a systematic review. *Sleep Medicine Review, 23C*, 10–19.

Morin, C.M., Leblanc, M., Bélanger, L., Ivers, H., Mérette, C. and Savard, J. (2011). Prevalence of insomnia and its treatment in Canada. *Canadian Journal of Psychiatry, 56*(9), 540–548. 10.1177/070674371105600905.

Nardi, P.M. (2014). *Doing Survey Research*, 3rd Ed. London: Paradigm Publishers.

National Sleep Foundation. (2019). Insomnia. Retrieved 11 December, 2019, from www.sleepfoundation.org/insomnia/what-causes-insomnia.

O'Connell, K. (2017). Effects of insomnia on the body. Retrieved 12 December, 2019, from www.healthline.com/health/insomnia-concerns.

Ota, A., Masue, T., Yasuda, N., Tsutsumi, A., Mino, Y., Ohara, H. and Ono, Y. (2009). Psychosocial job characteristics and insomnia: a prospective cohort study using the Demand-Control-Support (DCS) and Effort-Reward Imbalance (ERI) job stress models. *Sleep Medicine, 10*(10), 1112–1117.

Park, J. and Jung, M. (2009). A note on determination of sample size for a Likert scale. *Communications of the Korean Statistical Society, 16*(4), 669–673.

Paunio, T., Tuisku, K. and Korhonen, T. (2015). Sleep, work and mental health. *Psychiatria Fennica, 46*, 55–66.

Paunio, T., Korhonen, T., Hublin, C., Partinen, M., Kivimäki, M., Koskenvuo, M. and Kaprio, J. (2009). Longitudinal study on poor sleep and life dissatisfaction in a nationwide cohort of twins. *American Journal of Epidemiology, 169*(2), 206–213.

Pereira, D. and Elfering, A. (2014). Social stressors at work and sleep during weekends: The mediating role of psychological detachment. *Journal of Occupational Health Psychology*, *19*(1), 85–95. https://doi.org/10.1037/a0034928.

Reynolds, A.C., Appleton, S.L., Gill, T.K. and Adams, R.J. (2019). Chronic insomnia disorder in Australia. Retrieved 2 April, 2020, from www.sleephealthfoundation.org.au/pdfs/Special_Reports/SHF_Insomnia_Report_2019_Final_SHFlogo.pdf.

Riba, F.J. (1993). *Insomnia: Behavioural and Cognitive Interventions*. Geneva: World Health Organization – Division of Mental Health. https://apps.who.int/iris/handle/10665/58229.

Ribet, C. and Derriennic, F. (1999). Age, working conditions and sleep disorders: a longitudinal analysis in the French Cohort E.S.T.E.V. *Sleep*, *22*(4), 491–504.

Roth, T. (2007). Insomnia: definition, prevalence, etiology, and consequences. *Journal of Clinical Sleep Medicine: JCSM: Official publication of the American Academy of Sleep Medicine*, *3*(5 Suppl), S7–S10.

Salminen, S., Oksanen, T., Vahtera, J., Sallinen, M., Härmä, M., Salo, P., Virtanen, M. and Kivimäki, M. (2010). Sleep disturbances as a predictor of occupational injuries among public sector workers. *Journal of Sleep Research*, *19*(1 Pt 2), 207–213.

Salo, P., Ala-Mursula, L., Rod, N.H., Tucker, P., Pentti, J., Kivimäki, M. and Vahtera, J. (2014). Work time control and sleep disturbances: prospective cohort study of Finnish public sector employees. *Sleep*, *37*(7), 1217–1225.

Santos-Longhurst, A. (2018). What is chronic insomnia and how is it treated. Retrieved 11 December, 2019, from www.healthline.com/health/chronic-insomnia.

Scott, T.A. and Judge, P.A. (2006). Insomnia, emotions, and job satisfaction: a multilevel study. *Journal of Management*, *32*(5), 622–645.

Seixas, A., Ramos, A.R., Gordon-Strachan, G.M., Fonseca, V.A., Zizi, F. and Jean-Louis, G. (2014). Relationship between visual impairment, insomnia, anxiety/depressive symptoms among Russian immigrants. *Journal of Sleep Medicine and Disorders*, *1*(2), 1009.

Stranges, S., Dorn, J.M., Shipley, M.J., Kandala, N., Trevisan, M., Miller, M.A., Donahue, R.P., Hovey, K.M., Ferrie, J.E., Marmot, M.G. and Cappuccio, F.P. (2008). Correlates of short and long sleep duration: cross-cultural comparison between UK and US. The Whitehall II Study and the Western New York Health Study. *American Journal of Epidemiology*, *168*(12), 1353–1364.

Stranges, S., Tigbe, W., Gómez-Olivé, F.X., Thorogood, M. and Kandala, N.B. (2012). Sleep problems: an emerging global epidemic? Findings from the INDEPTH WHO-SAGE study among more than 40,000 older adults from 8 countries across Africa and Asia. *Sleep*, *35*(8), 1173–1181. https://doi.org/10.5665/sleep.2012.

Sutton, D.A., Moldofsky, H. and Badley, E.M. (2001). Insomnia and health problems in Canadians. *Sleep*, *24*, 665–670.

Swanson, M., Arnedt, J.T., Rosekind, M.R., Belenky, G., Balkin, T.J. and Drake, C. (2011). Sleep disorders and work performance: findings from the 2008 National Sleep Foundation Sleep in America poll. *Journal of Sleep Research*, *20*(3), 487–494.

Tenkanen, L., Sjöblom, T., Kalimo, R., Alikoski, T. and Härmä, M.I. (1997). Shift work, occupation and coronary heart disease over 6 years of follow-up in the Helsinki Heart Study. *Scandinavian Journal of Work, Environment and Health*, *23*(4), 257–265.

Van Laethem, M., Beckers, D.G.J., Kompier, M.A.J., Dijksterhuis, A.P. and Geurts, S.A.E. (2013). Psychosocial work characteristics and sleep quality: a systematic review of longitudinal and intervention research. *Scandinavian Journal of Work, Environment and Health*, *39*(6), 535–549.

Van Laethem, M., Beckers, D.G.J., Kompier, M.A.J., Kecklund, G., van den Bossche, S.N.J. and Geurts, S.A.E. (2015). Bidirectional relations between work-related stress, sleep quality and perseverative cognition. *Journal of Psychosomatic Research, 79*(5), 391–398.

WebMD. (2019). An overview of insomnia. Retrieved 10 December, 2019, from www.webmd.com/sleep-disorders/insomnia-causes#1.

Wijndaele, K., Matton, L., Duvigneaud, N., Lefevre, J., Bourdeaudhuij, I., Duquet, W., Thomis, M. and Philippaerts, R. (2007). Association between leisure time physical activity and stress, social support and coping: a cluster-analytical approach. *Psychology of Sport and Exercise, 8*(4), 425–440. 10.1016/j.psychsport.2006.08.001.

4 Work stress induced musculoskeletal disorders in construction

Work-related musculoskeletal disorders (WMSDs) are the most prevalent and costly health problem in the working population and account for 40% of work-related health cost globally (Punnett and Wegman 2004; Morken et al. 2003). Moreover, these health conditions are the most common cause of severe long-term pain, physical disability and loss of work. They also significantly affect the psychosocial status of affected people and their families (Woolf and Pfleger 2003). Due to their severity of consequences to affected employees and the number of employees affected by it, the Australian government has recognised WMSDs as priority disorders in the Australian Work Health and Safety Strategy 2012–2022. Other countries like the UK, USA, European Union countries and developed Asian nations also provide similar importance to them. WMSDs therefore warrant a priority in research studies too.

WMSDs have traditionally been associated with operatives and been believed to be caused by the impact of physical force or ergonomic issues at work. For example, the statistical summary produced by Safe Work Australia (2016) showed that all workers' compensations claimed for this category had body stressing and other physical hazards only as mechanisms for the incidents. Moreover, nearly 80% of the incidents were linked to operatives. However, recent research revealed that psychosocial conditions at work and job stress play an important role in the development of WMSDs.

In the construction industry too, WMSDs have largely been associated with operatives because of the scenario that only operatives are involved in physically strenuous activities. As a result, most research studies of WMSDs have focussed on physical factors, ergonomics and operatives in the construction industry. Given that the construction industry is notorious for job stress and with the evidence that job stress is a key cause of WMSDs, it is likely that a large proportion of construction professionals are also susceptible to WMSDs. Moreover, the workers' compensation system largely recognises only physical risk factors and mechanisms when assessing claims for WMSDs. This is owing to the wide availability and the acceptance of well-established epidemiological evidence on physical risk factors. It is paramount that a similar level of evidence is produced to lobby for recognition of job stress induced WMSDs too in the workers' compensation system. To that end, this chapter investigates job stress induced WMSDs among professionals in the Australian construction industry.

The remainder of the chapter is laid out as follows. An aetiological model of WMSDs is presented, followed by explanations of the research and analysis methods adopted. Then study findings are discussed, resulting in a new theory that models the relationships between job stressors, stress, WMSD and job performance. Finally, conclusions are drawn, highlighting key practical implications of the study.

Work-related musculoskeletal disorders (WMSDs)

Musculoskeletal disorders (MSDs) is an umbrella term for injuries or disorders of muscles, nerves, tendons, joints, cartilage and spinal discs in the human body. Work-related musculoskeletal disorders (WMSDs) are conditions in which the work environment and performance of work contribute significantly to the condition and/or the condition is made worse or persists longer due to work (Centers for Disease Control and Prevention 2018). Common types of WMSDs are (Korhan and Memon 2019):

- cervical vertebrae (symptom: neck pain/stiff neck)
- rotator cuff tendinitis (symptom: shoulder pain)
- lower back pain
- arthritis (pain, swelling and inflammation in and around the joints and other body organs)
- carpal tunnel syndrome (symptoms: numbness, tingling or burning sensation in the palms, fingers and wrists)
- elbow pain
- knee pain
- hernia.

American Psychological Association (2019) suggested that tension headaches and migraine headaches are also associated with muscle tension and may be grouped with WMSDs. These conditions are a result of musculoskeletal overstrain and are not associated with infectious, tumoral or general medical causes of inflammation that normally explain tissue lesions (Ministry of Social Affairs and Health 2015, cited in Roquelaure 2018).

Aetiology of WMSDs

Work-related musculoskeletal disorders were believed to be triggered primarily by biomechanical overstrain (body stressing). However, contemporary scientific literature identifies multi-factorial triggers, comprising occupational factors such as biomechanical/physical load, psychosocial stressors as well as personal factors such as demographic, medical conditions and psychological characteristics

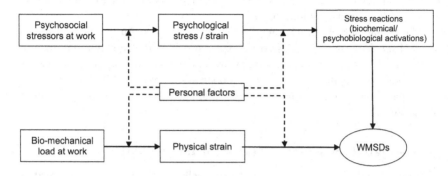

Figure 4.1 Model of the aetiology of WMSDs

(Roquelaure 2018). The model depicted in Figure 4.1 maps the aetiological pathway of WMSDs, which was derived from Stock et al. (2013), Hauke et al. (2011) and Carayon, Smith and Haims (1999), and the following sections explain the mechanisms in which these risk factors lead to WMSDs.

Biomechanical risk factors

Long existing epidemiological data prove that prolonged exposure to biomechanical loads at work is a major contributor to the onset of WMSDs and several risk factors at work have been reported under this category, which are (Korhan and Memon 2019; Roquelaure 2018; Kozak et al. 2015):

- highly repetitive movements (frequency, speed)
- intense efforts (force applied, weight carried/moved, general physical arduousness of working at the workstation)
- adoption of awkward postures for long periods (shoulder abduction, flexion/extension of the elbow or wrists, flexion/torsion of the torso)
- large range of movements
- using the heel of the palm or the elbow for support or localised pressure on these areas
- exposure to vibration
- working in cold conditions
- long exposure to physical constraints
- workstation ergonomics.

The biomechanical factors are more relevant to operatives who are involved in physical work and are less relevant to office-based employees. These have therefore been the primary focus of studies on WMSDs and related workers' compensation.

Psychosocial risk factors

American Psychological Association (2019) argued that job stress can cause musculoskeletal disorders. They further explained that at sudden onsets of mental stress, muscles tense up all at once as a natural guarding mechanism against danger, and then release the tension as the stress fades. Chronic stress causes the muscles to remain in a constant taut and tense state for long periods, triggering MSDs. This phenomenon was medically explained that the human body responds to stress via four systems that interact with the musculoskeletal system, which are: (1) arousal of the central nervous system, (2) activation of adrenal cortex (endocrine system), (3) activation of the secretion of cytokines by the immune system, and (4) activation of the vegetative nervous system (Hasenbring, Rusu and Turk 2012). Stress induced arousal of the central nervous system increases muscle tone, muscle stiffness and musculoskeletal load on the muscles and tendons, which raise the risks of MSDs (Schleifer et al. 2008; Eijckelhof et al. 2013; Taib, Bahn and Yun 2016). The central nervous system further activates the secretion of corticoids by the endocrine system and the release of pro-inflammatory cytokines. Corticoids may disturb the hydro-mineral balance of the body and increase sodium and fluid retention, which promotes the onset of tunnel syndromes (Palmer 2011; Aboonq 2015). Similarly, pro-inflammatory cytokines promote the onset of neuropathic tunnel pain and inflammatory tendon lesions in addition to impeding tendon tissue repair (Hasenbring, Rusu and Turk 2012; Burger, de Wet and Collins 2015; Millar, Murrell and McInnes 2017). Stress induced activation of the vegetative nervous system triggers the secretion of adrenaline and noradrenaline, which reduce microcirculation in the muscles and muscular tendons, resulting in: (1) reduced supply of nutrients to tendons, hindering its self-repair, and (2) early development of muscle fatigue and chronic muscle pain (Kumar 2007; Hasenbring, Rusu and Turk 2012; Davezies 2013 cited in Roquelaure 2018).

Numerous studies from around the world suggest that psychosocial risk factors at work result in job stress, which in turn leads to serious deterioration of mental and physical health of employees, including the onsets of WMSDs (European Agency for Safety and Health at Work 2007; Devereux et al. 2004; Canadian Centre for Occupational Health and Safety 2018; Safe Work Australia 2019). Table 4.1 presents these risks factors under nine categories. In addition to the risk factors shown in Table 4.1, the following have been reported in some other literature:

- Kim and Cho (2017) empirically assessed whether work–life conflict (WLC) is associated with WMSDs among Korean employees and discovered that WLC was significantly associated with an increased frequency of WMSDs in both men and women employees
- Clot (2015) and Davezies (2013, cited in Roquelaure et al. 2018) established a link between organisational injustice and WMSDs. Sara et al. (2018) defined organisational injustice as unfairness in the distribution of resources, the application of procedures and/or the treatment of employees with respect. In other words, this refers to discrimination in the workplace.

Table 4.1 Psychosocial risk factors linked to WMSDs

Category	Examples of psychosocial risk factors
Intensity and duration of work	• Work overload • Constraints related to work pace • Unrealistic or vague objectives • Excessive demands for adaptability • Contradictory instructions • Long working days, atypical work schedules, unpredictable working hours, etc. • Continually subject to deadlines
Job content	• Suitability of the task for the individual • Lack of variety or short work cycles • Fragmented or meaningless work • Exploitation
Emotional demands	• Expectation that emotions will be controlled and suppressed • Obligation to smile or pretend to be in a good mood • Conflict with members of the public, exposure to suffering or human stress • Full self-control in all circumstances and depicting a 'positive attitude' all times
Lack of autonomy	• Lack of agency over one's own work • Lack of decision-making freedom and room for manoeuvre (ability to organise one's own work) • Lack of employee involvement in decisions directly affecting their activities and the utilisation and development of their skills
Poor social relations at work	• Relations with colleagues and line managers • Work appraisal procedures • Value placed on employees' wellbeing • 'Pathologies' of social relations such as bullying
Lack of support and resources	• Lack of support for problem-solving • Lack of social support • Inadequate, unsuitable or unreliable resources for work
Conflicts of values	• Intra-psychological conflicts resulting from an imbalance between what is demanded at work and professional, social or personal values of employees
Job insecurity	• Socio-economic insecurity (fear of losing one's job, drop in wages, precarious contracts) • Risk of not being able to cope with changes to tasks and working conditions (restructuring, uncertainty about the future of one's job)
Career development	• Career stagnation • Under promotion or over promotion • Poor pay

Source: Adapted from Ministry of Labour, Employment and Health 2011 cited in Roquelaure 2018; Cox, Griffiths and Rial-Gonzalez 2000

Personal factors

Epidemiological evidence suggests that certain individual characteristics (age, gender, genetic dispositions) and medical conditions (obesity, diabetes, severe hypo-thyroidism, inflammatory rheumatism) increase the risk of developing WMSDs (Heilskov-Hansen et al. 2016; National Research Council 2001). However, Roquelaure (2018) cautioned that their impact should not be over-estimated; hence these may be considered confounding factors in WMSD onsets.

On the other hand, psychological literature suggests that personal psycho-logical characteristics have a profound impact on the subjective perception/ experience of stress and stress responses by individuals, thus constituting a highly personalised process and outcomes. Such characteristics include resili-ence, coping styles, perception and reappraisal (reframing) of stressful situations (cognitive reaction) and early experiences/exposure to stressful situations in life (Martin 2018; Lecic-Tosevski, Vukovic and Stepanovic 2011; Carayon, Smith and Haims 1999).

In summary, whilst the biomechanical load factors at work can be considered as direct causes of WMSDs, job stress caused by psychosocial stressors at work mediate biochemical/psychobiological changes in the body, eventually resulting in WMSDs. The biomechanical factors are more relevant to operatives who work on construction sites and less relevant to white-collar employees, but psychosocial risk factors are more pertinent to professionals. Personal factors such as demo-graphics, medical conditions and psychological characteristics act as confounding conditions and may produce individualised outcomes.

Research method

The model and the discussion presented in the preceding sections are of generic nature. Experiences and outcomes may vary depending on industry or employ-ment contexts. Hence, the remainder of the chapter investigates the situation in the Australian construction industry and experiments the utility of the WMSDs model presented in Figure 4.1. To this end, the following research questions are investigated empirically:

- What is the level of prevalence of WMSDs among construction professionals, and how does it vary due to socio-demographic factors?
- What are the most significant psychosocial risk factors that trigger WMSDs among construction professionals?
- How do individual stress coping styles affect WMSDs?
- How do the co-existence of work stress and stress coping styles predict WMSD outcomes?
- To what degree do WMSDs affect job outcomes among construction professionals?

Data

Data required for this study were collected through an online questionnaire survey in the Australian construction industry. Details of the questionnaire, survey administration and respondents were discussed in Chapter 1, and therefore are not repeated in this chapter, but the data subset applicable to this chapter is presented in Table 4.2. Moreover, a copy of the complete survey instrument can be found in the Appendix.

Table 4.2 Data pertinent to WMSDs

Section	Response options

Respondent's background
1. Gender (male, female or other)
2. Age (≤20, 21–30, 31–40, 41–50, 51–60 or >60)
3. Marital status (married/de-facto, single or divorced/separated/widowed)
4. Organisation type (property development, PM, architecture, engineering, QS, builder, subcontractor, FM or other)
5. Organisation size (measured by # of full-time employees) (≤4, 5–19, 20–199 or ≥200)
6. Job title (text responses were received but categorised as junior professional, mid-career professional, senior professional or executive)
7. Experience (<1 year, 1–5 years, 6–10 years or >10 years)
8. Nature of employment (permanent, fixed-term contract or casual)
9. Hours worked weekly (<20, 20–30, 30–40, 40–50 or >50)
10. Workplace environment (site or office)
11. Income (<$40k, $40–60k, $60–80k, $80–100k, $100–120k, $120–150k or >$150k)

Job stressors

In the past 6 months at work how often did you experience:

Measured using the scale of:
- Never
- Sometimes
- Often
- Always

1. Poor/dangerous work environment
2. Excessive workload
3. Unpredictable work hours
4. Time pressure
5. Job autonomy
6. Job appropriateness
7. Flexibility
8. Supportive feedback
9. Line manager support
10. Co-worker support
11. Harassment
12. Bullying
13. Discrimination
14. Role ambiguity
15. Adequate job resources
16. Staff consultation
17. Sufficient remuneration
18. Reward
19. Job security
20. Career prospect

Table 4.2 Cont.

Section	Response options
Work–private life conflict	
In the past 6 months how often did you experience:	Measured using the scale of:
1. Lack of energy for private life	• Never
2. Lack of time for private life	• Sometimes
3. Family complaint about too much work	• Often
4. Other personal life stressors	• Always
Chronic job stress	
In the past 4 weeks how often did you experience:	Measured using the scale of:
1. Poor sleep	• Never
2. Restlessness	• Sometimes
3. Irritability	• Often
4. Tensed	• Always
5. Nervousness	
Stress coping methods	
In the past 4 weeks how often did you engage in the following stress coping methods:	Measured using the scale of:
	• Not at all
1. Problem-solving	• Several days
2. Positive reappraisal	• More than half the days
3. Seeking support	• Nearly every day
4. Relaxation	
5. Physical activity	
6. Leisure and humour	
7. Eating balanced diet	
8. Adequate sleep	
9. Isolation	
10. Alcohol/drug use	
11. Smoking	
12. Emotional eating	
13. Criticise/blame others	
14. Compulsive spending	
15. Denial/ignoring as if nothing happened	
16. Releasing tension	
Musculoskeletal disorders	
A) In the past 6 months how often were you bothered by/treated for:	Measured using the scale of:
	• Never
1. Chronic headache/migraine	• Once or twice
2. Back, neck or shoulder pain	• Monthly
3. Arthritis	• Weekly
B) Do you believe that your job is the primary cause?	Dichotomous response –Yes / No
Job outcomes	
In the past 6 months how would you rate your:	Measured using a scale of 1 (low)
1. Job satisfaction	to 10 (high)
2. Job performance	

The survey was responded by 310 participants, but only 247 responses were complete and could be used for analysis. This was above the minimum required number of respondents, which is 241, for a survey that collects responses on a 4-point Likert scale with a 95% confidence level, as per Park and Jung (2009). Refer to Table 1.3 in Chapter 1 for socio-demographic details of the survey respondents. Except for the socio-demographic details of the respondents, responses to most other questions were collected on 4-point textural Likert scales, which were coded numerically in the following manner to facilitate quantitative analyses:

- Scale 1: never = 0, sometimes = 1, often = 2, always = 3
- Scale 2: not satisfied = 0, somewhat satisfied = 1, satisfied = 2, very satisfied = 3
- Scale 3: never = 0, once or twice = 1, monthly = 2, weekly = 3
- Scale 4: not at all = 0, several days = 1, more than half the days = 2, nearly every day = 3

Data analysis techniques

Various analysis techniques were used to answer the research questions as outlined here:

- The prevalence of WMSDs was assessed using descriptive statistics, along with inferential techniques such as one-sample t-tests for population. Moreover, Kruskal-Wallis H tests were performed to investigate how the differences in socio-economic factors influence WMSD experiences.
- Job stressors were grouped into suitable stressor constructs using Cronbach's alpha tests to facilitate analysis of interactions of stressors, coping styles, WMSDs and job outcomes.
- Correlation analyses were conducted to identify highly associated stress coping styles with WMSDs.
- Structural path analysis was performed to investigate the causal relationships between WMSDs and job stressor constructs and stress coping methods.

Construction professionals and WMSDs

This section discusses the analysis and findings under pertinent subsections.

Prevalence of WMSDs among construction professionals

Descriptive statistical analyses were conducted to understand the prevalence of WMSDs and their severity spread among construction industry professionals who responded to the survey. Participants' responses to the following two questions were studied:

A) In the past 6 months how often were you bothered by/treated for back, neck or shoulder pain?
   • Never
   • Once or twice
   • Monthly
   • Weekly

B) Do you believe that job stress may have caused this illness?
   • No
   • Yes

Three WMSDs were included in the survey, namely migraine or chronic headache, back, neck or shoulder pain, and arthritis. First, overall descriptive statistics were computed to identify the most prevalent condition that needs further scrutiny and Table 4.3 shows the results. Respondents rated the severity level on a 4-point Likert Scale (0–3: 0 = never bothered by/got treatment for; 3 = bothered by/got treatment for weekly). Though the literature identified numerous WMSD conditions, back, neck or shoulder pain appears to be the most prevalent condition among construction professionals. Hence, it is taken for further analysis in this chapter.

Around 57% of respondents indicated that they suffer from chronic back, neck or shoulder pain, but only 45% believed that this was induced by their work. Hence, to make further analysis robust, the 12% of responses that had indicated 'no' to the question whether it was caused by their job but suffered these conditions was removed from further consideration. Altogether 31 responses were filtered out. Then, one sample t-test was conducted on the filtered dataset to check whether the inferred population mean of 1.10 is significantly different from that of the sample that responded to the survey in this study. The results are shown in Figure 4.2 (a) to (c). The p-value of .159, which is greater than the threshold p-value of .05, suggests that the work stress induced back, neck or shoulder pain in the population of construction professionals is not significantly different from that of the sample surveyed. It can therefore be concluded that 45% of construction industry professionals in Australia suffer from work-related back, neck or shoulder pain and approximately 14% within the fraction receives treatment as frequently as once weekly.

The influence of socio-demographic factors such as gender, age, marital status, occupation level and organisation size on WMSDs was investigated using Kruskal-Wallis H tests. Kruskal-Wallis H test was chosen over ANOVA because the subgroups did not meet the normality and equal subsample size conditions. Table 4.4 presents the test results. Out of all five factors, only gender has an impact

Table 4.3 Descriptive statistics

WMSD condition	*Statistics*	
	Mean	*S*
Migraine or chronic headache	.50	.878
Back, neck or shoulder pain	1.02	1.074
Arthritis	.30	.781

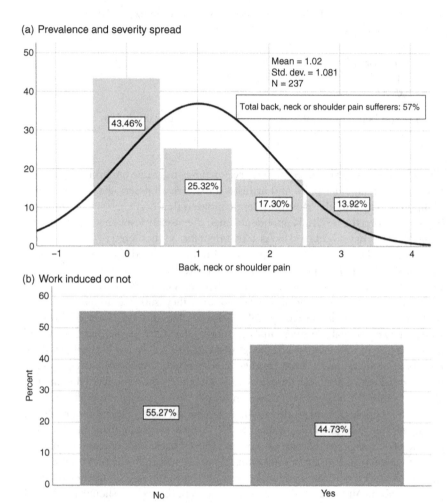

(a) Prevalence and severity spread

Mean = 1.02
Std. dev. = 1.081
N = 237

Total back, neck or shoulder pain sufferers: 57%

43.46%

25.32%

17.30%

13.92%

Back, neck or shoulder pain

(b) Work induced or not

Percent

55.27%

44.73%

No   Yes

Work induced back, neck or shoulder pain

(c) One sample t-test results

One-sample statistics				
	N	Mean	Std. deviation	Std. error mean
Back, neck or shoulder pain	216	.99	1.137	.077

One-sample test						
				Test value = 1.1		
			Sig.	Mean	95% Confidence interval of the difference	
	t	df	(2-tailed)	difference	Lower	Upper
Back, neck or shoulder pain	−1.412	215	.159	−.109	−.26	.04

Figure 4.2 Prevalence of back, neck or shoulder pains

Table 4.4 Influence of socio-demographic factors on WMSDs

Factor		N	Mean Rank	Null hypothesis	Kruskal-Wallis H	Sig	Decision
Gender	Male	165	102.85	WMSD experiences are the same across different genders of professionals	6.599	.037	**Reject null hypothesis**
	Female	48	126.75				
	Other	3	127.50				
Age	Below 20	1	199.50	WMSD experiences are the same across different age categories of professionals	3.046	.693	Retain null hypothesis
	20 to 30	69	110.93				
	31 to 40	52	104.94				
	41 to 50	53	106.07				
	51 to 60	26	112.69				
	Over 60	15	104.90				
Marital status	Married/de-facto	142	111.60	WMSD experiences are the same across professionals with different marital status	3.551	.470	Retain null hypothesis
	Never married	59	103.19				
	Separated	8	117.75				
	Widowed	6	72.00				
	Unspecified	1	126.50				
Occupation level	Junior	56	99.94	WMSD experiences are the same across different occupational levels of professionals	1.365	.714	Retain null hypothesis
	Mid-career	51	109.63				
	Senior	71	110.01				
	Executive	33	102.05				
Organisation size	Employees ≤4	18	112.44	WMSD experiences are the same across professionals from different sizes of organisation	1.283	.733	Retain null hypothesis
	5 to 19	42	101.49				
	20 to 199	68	113.23				
	Employees ≥200	87	106.14				

on WMSDs among construction professionals as demonstrated by the p-value of less than .05. The mean rank values further suggest that female professionals suffer more from WMSDs than their counterpart.

Epidemiological literature suggests that age and gender increase the risk of developing WMSDs (Heilskov-Hansen et al. 2016; National Research Council 2001) though Roquelaure (2018) cautioned that their impact is not significant. This study found that gender has a statistically significant influence in WMSDs whilst age did not reveal a remarkable influence.

Predictors of WMSDs

The role of job stress and stress coping styles of individuals in predicting WMSDs is analysed in this section. The survey contained 22 job stressors and 16 stress coping methods. In order to simplify the analysis, job stressors and stress coping styles were first organised suitable constructs. Following that the interactions of the constructs in predicting WMSDs are analysed using a structural path model.

Establishing constructs for job stressors

The identification of constructs and assigning relevant stressors under them were guided by well-tried and tested existing theories and previous research. Hence, dimension reduction or exploratory factor analysis from first principles was not performed. Rather, in order to ensure that the measurement items (assigned stressors) adequately represent the constructs, internal consistency and reliability tests were conducted using Cronbach's α tests. Moreover, the connotational directional manner in which the questions were worded for stressors was also considered when grouping stressors (please see the questionnaire in the Appendix for the wording of stressors). Stressors that were worded in the same connotational direction were only combined in the constructs. Some stressors were removed from further considerations, based on the Cronbach's α analysis results. Moreover, statistical means were computed for grouped stressors (constructs) for use in further analyses. Table 4.5 depicts the results. To accept that a construct is reliable and the measurement items within a construct are internally consistent, the Cronbach's α value of above .70 is preferred (Tavakol and Dennick 2011), though there are debates in the literature over what is the acceptable lowest value. In Table 4.5, however, the construct 'job resources' has a value of .671. It was essential to combine only stressors that were assessed with the same directional statements. Moreover, there were only two relevant stressors that can be grouped under this construct. Nonetheless, the yielded alpha for the construct is only marginally below .70.

Table 4.5 Constructs of job stressors

Construct	Job stressors	Cronbach's α	Mean
High job demand	• Excessive workload • Unpredictable work hours • Excessive time pressure	.791	1.379
Job control & support	• Autonomy • Flexibility with time • Supportive feedback • Line manager support • Co-worker support	.709	1.781
Workplace injustice	• Harassment • Bullying	.762	1.675
Job resources	• Role clarity • Resources	.671	.300
Job rewards	• Sufficient remuneration • Recognition • Job security • Career prospect	.774	1.766
Work–life conflict	• Lack of energy for private life • Lack of time for private life • Family complaint about too much work • Other personal life stressors	.826	1.275
Work stress	• Poor sleep • Restlessness • Irritability • Tensed • Nervousness	.919	1.178

Significant stressor constructs and stress coping styles

In a bid to further reduce the variables considered for causal analysis, Pearson correlation analyses were performed to identify stress constructs and stress coping styles that are significantly associated with WMSDs. Table 4.6 presents the correlation results for stressor constructs. It is evident that all stressor constructs are significantly correlated with back, neck or shoulder pain experienced by construction professionals though with varying strengths. Work–life conflict, high job demand and job resources are more strongly correlated than job rewards, job control and support, and workplace injustice, which show negative correlation. Table 4.7 shows the correlations between stress coping styles and back, neck or shoulder pain experiences. Only half of the 16 coping methods are significantly correlated and out of these eight styles, only five yielded correlation coefficients close to .30, which are emotional eating, blaming others, numbing, releasing tension and compulsive spending. Coefficients for other coping methods are significantly smaller than .30, which makes the value the threshold for accepting coping methods for further analysis. All these are maladaptive coping styles. Hence, a single construct

Table 4.6 Correlations between stressor constructs and WMSDs

Stressor construct	Back, neck or shoulder pain	
	Correlation coefficient	Sig. (2-tailed)
High job demand	.229**	.000
High job control and support	−.153*	.016
Workplace injustice	−.145*	.023
Job resources	.204**	.001
Job rewards	−.184**	.004
Work–life conflict	.246**	.000

** Correlation is significant at the .01 level (2-tailed).
* Correlation is significant at the .05 level (2-tailed).

Table 4.7 Correlations between stress coping styles and WMSDs

Stress coping style	Back, neck or shoulder pain	
	Correlation coefficient	Sig. (2 tailed)
Problem-solving	.138*	.037
Keeping a positive attitude	−.101	.127
Seeking external support	.185**	.005
Relaxation	.021	.756
Physical activity	.029	.667
Engaged in humour, fun and leisure activities	.014	.835
Eating well-balanced meals	.035	.594
Resting and sleeping enough	−.087	.192
Escape – isolating from others	.119	.073
Numbing – consuming alcohol or drugs	.287**	.000
Smoking to get a relief from stress	.094	.157
Emotional eating and drinking	.301**	.000
Criticising or blaming others for the situation	.298**	.000
Compulsive spending	.225**	.001
Ignoring as if nothing happened (denial/ distancing)	.131*	.048
Releasing tension	.260**	.000

** Correlation is significant at the .01 level (2-tailed).
* Correlation is significant at the .05 level (2-tailed).

was formed by combining these five styles to represent in further analyses, namely maladaptive coping. Akin to stressor constructs, a Cronbach α test was performed to test the internal validity of the construct, which yielded an α value of .758.

Structural path analysis

Figure 4.3 conceptualises the causal relationship between job stressor constructs and WMSDs, which has been derived from the literature discussed in the preceding

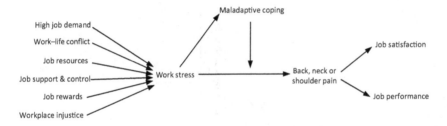

Figure 4.3 Causal pathway between stressors and WMSDs

sections. It theorises that encountering job stressors results in work stress, which in turn causes WMSDs, particularly back, neck or shoulder pain. Additionally, work stress may trigger maladaptive coping habits in construction professionals and the causal relationship between work stress and WMSDs is escalated by the maladaptive coping. Subsequently, experiences of chronic back, neck or shoulder pain diminish job satisfaction and performance levels.

The hypothesised cause and effect relationships were tested using structural path analysis on IBM AMOS 26. Path modelling was preferred over multiple regression or hierarchical multiple regression because it allows the examination of a series of cause and effect relationships simultaneously (Hair et at. 2014). This is particularly relevant to the present context because the hypothesised model consists of multiple regression equations.

The conceptual model shown in Figure 4.3 was replicated in the AMOS graphical interface and model testing was conducted using the survey data in an iterative manner until a best fitting model for the dataset was achieved. Modification indices suggested by AMOS were used in remodelling. After many iterations, the model shown in Figure 4.4 yielded acceptable model fit statistics. The resultant model is slightly different from the conceptual model illustrated in Figure 4.3. Modifications by eliminating the effects on job outcomes were required to achieve a best fitting model. The next paragraphs discuss the statistical parameters derived from the analysis for the final model.

Schumacker and Lomax (2015) provided a guideline for assessing model fitness, as shown in Table 4.8. The path model presented earlier yielded the following fitness values: CFI = .997, TLI = 1.014, NFI = .993, and RMSEA = .000. A value close to 1 for CFI, TLI and NFI as well as a value close to 0 for RMSEA suggests a good model fit. It is therefore concluded that the model presented in Figure 4.4 fits the dataset well. Respective regression weights for the paths, squared multiple correlations (R^2), associated levels of significance (p-values) and intercepts are shown in Figure 4.4 and Table 4.9.

Several statistically significant direct pathways (effects) were identified in the path analysis. Work–life conflict ($\beta = .505$, p <.01), high job demand ($\beta = .229$, p <.01) and job control and support ($\beta = -.154$, p =.005) are significant predictors of work stress that induce WMSDs. However, workplace injustice ($\beta = -.038$,

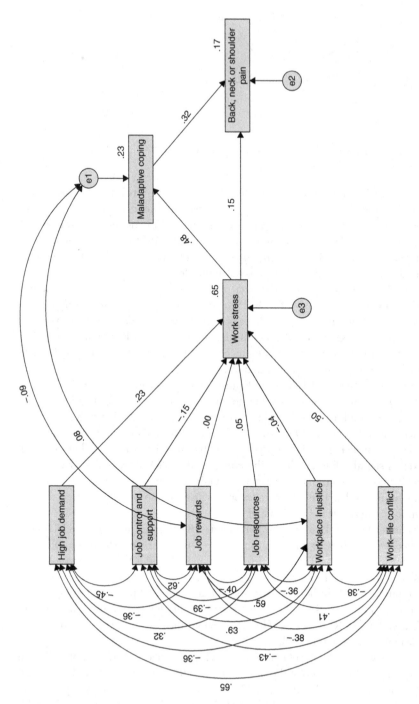

Figure 4.4 Path model of work stress induced back, neck or shoulder pain

Table 4.8 Model fit criteria for path models (Schumacker and Lomax 2015, p112)

Model fit criterion	Acceptable level	Interpretation
Chi-square (χ^2)	Tabled χ^2 value	Compares obtained χ^2 value with tabled value for given *df*
Goodness-of-fit index (GFI)	0 (no fit) to 1 (perfect fit)	Value close to .90 or .95 reflects a good fit
Adjusted GFI	0 (no fit) to 1 (perfect fit)	Value adjusted for *df*, with .90 or .95 a good model fit
Root-mean square residual (RMR)	Researcher defines level	Indicates the closeness of Σ to S matrices
Standardised RMS (SRMR)	< .05	Value less than .05 indicates a good model fit
Root mean square error of approximation (RMSEA)	.05 to .08	Value of .05 to .08 indicates close fit
Tucker-Lewis Index (TLI)	0 (no fit) to 1 (perfect fit)	Value close to .90 or .95 reflects a good model fit
Normed fit index (NFI)	0 (no fit) to 1 (perfect fit)	Value close to .90 or .95 reflects a good model fit
Parsimony fit index (PNFI)	0 (no fit) to 1 (perfect fit)	Compares values in alternative models
Akaike information criterion (AIC)	0 (perfect fit) to positive value (poor fit)	Compares values in alternative models

Table 4.9 Regression weights of direct effects and intercepts

Direct predictor relationship	Standardised regression weight	p-value
High job demand → Work stress	.229	***
Job control & support → Work stress	−.154	.005
Workplace injustice → Work stress	−.038	.463
Job resources → Work stress	.054	.212
Job rewards → Work stress	.002	.977
Work life conflict → Work stress	.505	***
Work stress → Maladaptive coping	.478	***
Work stress → Back, neck or shoulder pain	.151	.022
Maladaptive coping → Back, neck or shoulder pain	.321	***
	Intercept	
e1	.280	***
e2	.951	***
e3	.174	***

p =.463), job resources (β = −.054, p = .212) and job rewards (β = .002, p = .977) were not found to have significant direct effects. Work stress triggers maladaptive coping habits such as numbing, emotional eating, releasing tension, blaming and compulsive spending, which appear to be confounders of WMSDs, with

$\beta = .478$ and p < .01. Similarly, work stress ($\beta = .151$, p = .022) and maladaptive coping habits ($\beta = .321$, p < .01) are significant predictors of WMSDs, particularly back, neck or shoulder pain among construction professionals. Based on the findings, the following equations can be formulated to explain the cause and effect relationships:

WMSDs = .15 x Work stress + .32 x Maladaptive coping + .951

Maladaptive coping = .48 x Work stress + .280

Work stress = .50 x Work–life conflict + .23 x high job demand + .174

Table 4.10 illustrates correlation estimates between stressor constructs. Two statistically significant predictors of work stress such as high job demand and work–life conflict appear to be highly correlated positively (correlation coefficient = .653). High job demand is characterised in this research as a combination of excessive workload, unpredictable work hours and excessive work hours. It is apparent that such characteristics of one's job are likely to accumulate unfulfilled family responsibilities, stress and thereby experiences of WMSDs.

In summary, the study finds that work stress induced back, neck or shoulder pain among construction professionals is triggered largely by job stressors such as excessive workload, unpredictable work hours, excessive work hours and work–life conflict. The pain experiences worsen when the construction professional adopts stress coping styles such as numbing (consuming alcohol/drugs), emotional eating and drinking (consuming comfort food and caffeine drinks), releasing tension by

Table 4.10 Correlations between stressor constructs

Correlations	Estimate
Job control & support <–> High job demand	−.448
Workplace injustice <–> High job demand	−.360
Job resources <–> High job demand	.315
Job rewards <–> High job demand	−.358
Work–life conflict <–> High job demand	.653
Job control & support <–> Workplace injustice	.627
Job control & support <–> Job resources	−.387
Job control & support <–>Job rewards	.623
Job control & support <–>Work–life conflict	−.435
Workplace injustice <–> Work–life conflict	−.379
Job resources <–> Work–life conflict	.411
Job rewards <–> Work–life conflict	−.379
Workplace injustice <–> Job resources	−.361
Job resources <–> Job rewards	−.401
Workplace injustice <–> Job rewards	.585
e1<–>Workplace injustice	.079
e1<–>Job rewards	−.088

crying, yelling or throwing things, blaming others for the situation, and/or compulsive spending (shopping/buying gifts for oneself frequently to feel happy). Moreover, construction professionals' job performance and satisfaction levels do not seem to be affected significantly by the experiences of work stress induced back, neck or shoulder pain.

Discussion

The findings of this study confirm some previous studies whilst contradicting some others found in both construction and general occupational epidemiology.

Leung, Chan and Dongyu (2011) and Leung, Chan and Cooper (2015) reported that construction professionals in Hong Kong were susceptible to headaches, migraines and back pain due to work stress. They further found that musculoskeletal (i.e. back, neck or shoulder) pain was more prevalent than other types of diseases that are induced by work stress, including headaches and migraines. This study confirms that in the context of the Australian construction industry also the prevalence of back, neck or shoulder pain is higher than headaches and migraines. Leung, Chan and Cooper (2015) compared the experiences of musculoskeletal pain across different occupational, age and gender categories and asserted that quantity surveyors who are generally junior to mid-career professional category reported higher musculoskeletal pains though they do not generally work on site. However, they often tend to have a substantial amount of estimating work and work long hours constantly, which may be responsible for the pain experiences (Leung, Chan and Cooper 2015). The current study contradicts the former assertion whilst agreeing with the latter. The study did not find any statistically significant differences across different occupational levels (see Table 4.4). The study further reveals that high volume of work and excessive work hours are significant triggers of work stress and therefore WMSDs. Leung, Chan and Cooper (2015) further claimed that there were no statistically significant differences in the experience of musculoskeletal pain due to the age or gender of construction professionals. This study agrees with the former but disagrees with the latter in the Australian context, whereby female professionals experience higher levels of back, neck or shoulder pain.

The aetiological model discussed in the earlier part of the chapter argued that biochemical changes that happen in the body due to stress are the primary trigger of WMSDs. In other words, poor psychosocial conditions at work directly influence the onset of WMSDs. Micheletti et al. (2019), however, claimed that there is a close association between lifestyle factors such as physical activity during leisure, smoking, alcohol intake and unhealthy eating, and musculoskeletal pain intensity in the lower back, neck or shoulder in the working population. However, less is known about the role of maladaptive coping habits and lifestyle adopted by individuals in the WMSD aetiology. The present study reveals that lifestyle factors – such as emotional eating and drinking, alcohol or drug consumption, aggressive reactions like blaming others and releasing tension by yelling as well as compulsive buying – exacerbate WMSDs. This relationship is clinically explained and supported by the literature in epidemiology as explained in the ensuing paragraph.

Mierswa and Kellmann (2017) showed an increased risk of developing low back pain among university administrative employees who were smokers. Similarly, Ferreira et al. (2013) claimed that alcohol addiction was associated with complex and chronic low back pain. The current study claims that alcohol and/or drug consumption predicts back, neck or shoulder pain, but no significant association is found between these diseases and smoking among construction professionals in Australia. Bohman et al. (2014) asserted that the consumption of fruits and vegetables along with other healthy behaviour was associated with the prognosis of lower back pain. The current study finds the reverse to be confirmed that consumption of unhealthy food and drinks whilst confronted with work stress predicts the diagnosis of back, neck or shoulder pain. Tilov et al. (2016) studied the relationship between one's psychological character, such as aggression, and chronic diseases. They concluded that there was a statistically significant relationship between psychological character such as anger, hostility in patients and chronic diseases such as diabetes, hypertension and musculoskeletal disorders. The present study reveals that aggressive reactions such as blaming others or releasing tension by yelling or throwing things predict WMSDs. The present study found compulsive spending/buying to be a prominent maladaptive stress coping behaviour that predicts WMSDs. It seems difficult to see a causal connection between buying habits and WMSDs. Nonetheless, Zhang et al. (2016) explained that compulsive buying and substance (alcohol/drug) dependency are closely associated. Hence, it can be deduced that consuming alcohol or drugs to forget work stress triggers compulsive behaviour patterns in construction professionals.

All in all, the present study adds a new perspective and knowledge to the aetiology of work-related musculoskeletal disorders by identifying dominant predictors from job stressors and lifestyle factors. It also strengthens some existing literature both in construction and occupational epidemiology.

Conclusion

Work-related musculoskeletal disorders (WMSDs) are the most prevalent and costly health concern in the working population, accounting for 40% of the work-related health cost globally. They are also classified as priority disorders by the governments in many developed countries, including Australia. Traditionally, physical force/body stressing and ergonomic issues at work have been regarded as the primary causes of WMSDs, and as such they have been associated largely with operatives in the construction industry. Nonetheless, recent evidence from the epidemiological literature suggests that work stress is a major cause of WMSDs. It is well-established through sound research that construction professionals are enduring excessive work stress globally. It is therefore likely that a large proportion of them suffer from WMSDs. Yet, this has never been explored in detail before.

Through robust research and analysis, this study revealed several key insights related to WMSDs among construction professionals in Australia.

Forty-five percent of construction industry professionals in Australia suffer from work stress induced back, neck or shoulder pain and one-third of them receive treatment as frequently as weekly. Moreover, female professionals suffer more frequently than their counterpart. Work–life conflict and excessive job demand, caused by heavy workload, unpredictable and long work hours, are the primary determinants. Excessive job demand is also a contributor to work–life conflict. Moreover, stress induced by these factors triggers certain maladaptive stress coping habits that contribute to WMSDs as well. Alarming maladaptive coping habits are emotional eating and drinking, alcohol or drug consumption, aggressive reactions like blaming others and/or releasing tension by yelling as well as compulsive behaviour like addictive buying/shopping.

There are few significant practical implications from these findings for the insurance scheme, the construction industry and construction professionals. Traditionally, body stressing/physical force has been largely considered as an acceptable cause for WMSDs in workers' compensation claims. However, evidence from the present study proves that work stress is also a significant cause of WMSDs and therefore the assessment of risk factors for WMSDs should be broadened to include work stress. The construction industry altogether should make some adjustments to the current norms around volume of work and work hours to reduce its footprint in the global statistics of WMSDs. This is also a necessary adjustment for building healthy, sustainable families and communities. Female professionals should be prioritised in receiving the benefits of such adjustments since they are worse affected by WMSDs. Individual construction professionals should adopt a healthy lifestyle and habits to manage work stress though these might require extra efforts and take longer to produce positive effects. Such a lifestyle is characterised by regular physical exercise, healthy diet, regular leisure activities and adequate relaxation and sleep. At the workplace, communications with colleagues to solve problems and seeking support is encouraged to curtail stressors. Shortcut measures such as emotional eating, alcohol/drug intake or aggressive responses may seem to provide a quick fix and relief but in fact they worsen mental and physical health.

References

Aboonq, M.S. (2015). Pathophysiology of carpal tunnel syndrome. *Neurosciences*, *20*(1), 4–9.

American Psychological Association. (2019). Stress effects on the body. Retrieved 19 August, 2019, from www.apa.org/helpcenter/stress-body.

Bohman, T., Alfredsson, L., Jensen, I., Hallqvist, J., Vingård, E. and Skillgate, E. (2014). Does a healthy lifestyle behaviour influence the prognosis of low back pain among men and women in a general population? A population-based cohort study. *BMJ Open*, *4*(12), e005713.

Burger, M.C., de Wet, H. and Collins, M. (2015). Interleukin and growth factor gene variants and risk of carpal tunnel syndrome. *Gene*, *564*(1), 67–72.

Canadian Centre for Occupational Health and Safety. (2018). Mental health – psychosocial risk factors in the workplace. Retrieved 17 October, 2019, from www.ccohs.ca/oshanswers/psychosocial/mentalhealth_risk.html.

Carayon, P., Smith, M.J. and Haims, M.C. (1999). Work organization, job stress, and workrelated musculoskeletal disorders. *Human Factors, 41*(4), 644–663.

Centers for Disease Control and Prevention. (2018). Work-related musculoskeletal disorders and ergonomics. Retrieved 16 October, 2019, from www.cdc.gov/workplace healthpromotion/health-strategies/musculoskeletal-disorders/index.html.

Clot, Y. (2015). *La fonction psychologique du travail.* Paris: PUF.

Cox, T., Griffiths, A. and Rial-Gonzalez, E. (2000). *Work-Related Stress.* Luxembourg: Office for Official Publications of the European Communities.

Devereux, J., Rydstedt, L., Kelly, V., Weston, P. and Buckle, P. (2004). The role of work stress and psychological factors in the development of musculoskeletal disorders: the stress and MSD study. HSE Research Report 273, Robens Centre for Health Ergonomics, Guildford, Surrey.

Eijckelhof, B.H., Huysmans, M.A., Garza, J.L.B., Blatter, B.M., van Dieën, J.H., Dennerlein, J.T. and van der Beek, A.J. (2013). The effects of workplace stressors on muscle activity in the neck-shoulder and forearm muscles during computer work: a systematic review and meta-analysis. *European Journal of Applied Physiology, 113*(12), 2897–2912.

European Agency for Safety and Health at Work. (2007). Expert forecast on emerging psychosocial risks related to occupational safety and health. Retrieved 22 October, 2019, from https://osha.europa.eu/en/publications/report-expert-forecast-emerging-psychosocial-risks-related-occupational-safety-and.

Ferreira, P.H., Pinheiro, M.B., Machado, G.C. and Ferreira, M.L. (2013). Is alcohol intake associated with low back pain? A systematic review of observational studies. *Manual Therapy, 18*(3), 183–190.

Hair, J.F., Black, W.C., Babin, B.J. and Anderson, R.E. (2014). *Multivariate Data Analysis,* 7th Ed. Harlow: Pearson Education Limited.

Hasenbring, M.I., Rusu, A.C. and Turk, D.C. (2012). *From Acute to Chronic Back Pain: Risk Factors, Mechanisms, and Clinical Implications.* Oxford: Oxford University Press.

Hauke, A., Flintrop, J., Brun, E. and Rugulies, R. (2011). The impact of work-related psychosocial stressors on the onset of musculoskeletal disorders in specific body regions: a review and meta-analysis of 54 longitudinal studies. *Work Stress, 25*(3), 243–256.

Heilskov-Hansen, T., Mikkelsen, S., Svendsen S.W., Thygesen, L.C., Hansson, G. and Thomsen, J.F. (2016). Exposure-response relationships between movements and postures of the wrist and carpal tunnel syndrome among male and female house painters: a retrospective cohort study. *Occupational and Environmental Medicine, 73*(6), 401–408.

Kim, Y.M. and Cho, S.I. (2017). Work-life imbalance and musculoskeletal disorders among South Korean workers. *International Journal of Environmental Research and Public Health, 14*(11), pii:1331. doi: 10.3390/ijerph14111331.

Korhan, O. and Memon, A.A. (2019). Introductory chapter: work-related musculoskeletal disorders. Retrieved 15 August, 2019, from www.intechopen.com/books/work-related-musculoskeletal-disorders/introductory-chapter-work-related-musculoskeletal-disorders.

Kozak, A., Schedlbauer, G., Wirth, T., Euler, U., Westermann, C. and Nienhaus, A. (2015). Association between work-related biomechanical risk factors and the occurrence of carpal tunnel syndrome: an overview of systematic reviews and a meta-analysis of current research. *BMC Musculoskeletal Disorders, 16*(1), 231.

Kumar, S. (eds.) (2007). *Biomechanics in Ergonomics,* 2nd ed., Boca Raton: CRC Press.

Lecic-Tosevski, D., Vukovic, O. and Stepanovic, J. (2011). Stress and personality. *Psychiatriki*, *22*(4), 290–297.

Leung, M., Chan, I.Y.S. and Cooper, C.L. (2015). *Stress Management in the Construction Industry*. West Sussex, UK: Wiley Blackwell.

Leung, M., Chan, Y.S.I. and Dongyu, C. (2011). Structural linear relationships between job stress, burnout, physiological stress, and performance of construction project managers. *Engineering, Construction and Architectural Management*, *18*(3), 312–328.

Martin, B. (2018). Stress and personality. *Psych Central*. Retrieved 18 October, 2019, from https://psychcentral.com/lib/stress-and-personality/.

Micheletti, J.K., Bláfoss, R., Sundstrup, E., Bay, H., Pastre, C.M. and Andersen, L.L. (2019). Association between lifestyle and musculoskeletal pain: cross-sectional study among 10,000 adults from the general working population. *BMC Musculoskeletal Disorders*, *20*, 609. https://doi.org/10.1186/s12891-019-3002-5.

Mierswa, T. and Kellmann, M. (2017). Psychological detachment as moderator between psychosocial work conditions and low back pain development. *International Journal of Occupational Medicine and Environmental Health*, *30*(2), 313–327.

Millar, N.L., Murrell, G.A. and McInnes, I.B. (2017). Inflammatory mechanisms in tendinopathy: towards translation, Nature Reviews. *Rheumatology*, *13*(2), 110–122.

Morken, T., Riise, T., Moen, B., Hauge, S.H.V., Holien, S., Langedrag, A., Pedersen, S., Saue, I.L.L., Seljebø, G.M. and Thoppil, V. (2003). Low back pain and widespread pain predict sickness absence among industrial workers. *BMC Musculoskeletal Disorders*, *4*, 21. doi: 10.1186/1471-2474-4-21.

National Research Council. (2001). *Musculoskeletal Disorders and the Workplace: Low Back and Upper Extremities*. Washington, DC: National Academy Press.

Palmer, K.T. (2011). Carpal tunnel syndrome: the role of occupational factors, Best Practice and Research. *Clinical Rheumatology*, *25*(1), 15–29.

Park, J. and Jung, M. (2009). A note on determination of sample size for a Likert scale. *Communications of the Korean Statistical Society*, *16*(4), 669–673.

Punnett, L. and Wegman D.H. (2004). Work-related musculoskeletal disorders: the epidemiologic evidence and the debate. *Journal of Electromyography and Kinesiology*, *14*, 13–23. doi: 10.1016/j.jelekin.2003.09.015.

Roquelaure, Y. (2018). Musculoskeletal disorders and psychosocial factors at work. *European Trade Union Institute Report*, *142*. Brussels: UTUI aisbl.

Safe Work Australia. (2016). Statistics on work-related musculoskeletal disorders. Retrieved 16 October, 2019, from www.safeworkaustralia.gov.au/system/files/documents/1702/statistics_on_work-related_musculoskeletal_disorders.pdf.

Safe Work Australia. (2019). Mental health. Retrieved 17 October, 2019, from www.safeworkaustralia.gov.au/topic/mental-health.

Sara, J.D., Prasad, M., Eleid, M.F., Zhang, M., Widmer, R.J. and Lerman, A. (2018). Association between work-related stress and coronary heart disease: a review of prospective studies through the job strain, effort-reward balance, and organizational justice models. *Journal of the American Heart Association*, *7*(9), e008073. doi:10.1161/JAHA.117.008073.

Schleifer, L.M., Spalding, T.W., Kerick, S.E., Cram, J.R., Ley, R. and Hatfield, B.D. (2008). Mental stress and trapezius muscle activation under psychomotor challenge: a focus on EMG gaps during computer work. *Psychophysiology*, *45*(3), 356–365.

Schumacker, R.E. and Lomax, R.G. (2015). *A Beginner's Guide to Structural Equation Modelling*, 4th ed. New York and London: Routledge.

Stock, S., Nicolakakis, N., Messing, K., Turcot, A. and Raiq, H. (2013). What is the relation between work-related musculoskeletal disorders and psychosocial factors? An overview of various conceptualizations of psychosocial work factors and proposal of a new model of MSD development. PISTES; 15-2.

Taib, M.F., Bahn, S. and Yun, M.H. (2016). The effect of psychosocial stress on muscle activity during computer work: comparative study between desktop computer and mobile computing products, Work. *A Journal of Prevention, Assessment, and Rehabilitation, 54*(3), 543–555.

Tavakol, M. and Dennick, R. (2011). Making sense of Cronbach's alpha. *International Journal of Medical Education, 2,* 53–55. https://doi.org/10.5116/ijme.4dfb.8dfd

Tilov, B., Semerdzhieva, M., Bakova, D., Tornyova, B. and Stoyanov, D. (2016). Study of the relationship between aggression and chronic diseases (diabetes and hypertension). *Journal of Evaluation in Clinical Practice, 22*(3), 421–424.

Woolf, A.D. and Pfleger, B. (2003). Burden of major musculoskeletal conditions. *Bulletin of the World Health Organisation, 81*(9), 646–656.

Zhang, C., Brook, J.S., Leukefeld, C.G. and Brook, D.W. (2016). Associations between compulsive buying and substance dependence/abuse, major depressive episode, and generalized anxiety disorder among men and women. *Journal of Addictive Diseases, 35*(4), 298–304.

5 Work stress induced weight gain in construction

World Health Organization (WHO) (2018) defined overweight and obesity as abnormal or excessive fat accumulation in the body that may impair health. It is commonly measured by body mass index (BMI), a ratio of weight-to-height of a person, in which the weight in kilograms is divided by the square of the height (kg/m^2). An individual with a BMI ≥ 25 is classified overweight whilst the one with a BMI ≥ 30 is considered obese. Ritchie and Roser (2019) claimed that 13% of adults in the world today are obese and another 39% are overweight. Australian Institute of Health and Welfare (2019) warned that overweight, particularly obesity, increases the risk of type 2 diabetes, cardiovascular disorders, musculo-skeletal disorders and certain cancers. Obesity is also a leading risk factor for early death; 4.7 million global deaths (8%) were linked to obesity in 2017 (Ritchie and Roser 2019).

Public health literature argues that the primary cause of overweight and obesity is an imbalance between calories consumed and spent, which is a result of the combination of an increased consumption of calorie-dense food and an increased physical inactivity due to a sedentary lifestyle. Nonetheless, recently, researchers have claimed that stress, including work stress, is a significant risk factor for over-weight and obesity. Traditionally, obesity or overweight has not been considered as a work health and safety (WHS) issue but recent evidence shows strong asso-ciations between obesity/overweight and psychosocial work factors such as long work hours, shift work, job demands, job control, role conflict, leadership quality, job insecurity, organisational culture and social support (Poulsen et al. 2014; Solovieva et al. 2013).

Construction being notorious for work stress and poor psychosocial work conditions, construction professionals may be at high risk of overweight and obesity and subsequent complications. However, this is an unexplored topic in construction management literature. Hence, this chapter investigates work stress induced weight gain among construction professionals in Australia, its risk factors, and job and health consequences. The chapter is organised as follows. First, epi-demiological reasoning behind the relationship between work stress and weight gain is elucidated. Then, the research method adopted to achieve the aim of this chapter is explained. Following that the research findings are expounded. Finally, the chapter is concluded with insights for practical implications.

Work stress to obesity

Figure 5.1 explains the pathway that connects work stress, and overweight and obesity. Enduring persistent job stressors triggers work stress, which in turn activates three types of responses in the human body that mediate rapid, excessive weight gains, leading to more serious health complications such as diabetes, cardiovascular disorders, musculoskeletal disorders and certain cancers. The responses to work stress are related to physiology, behaviour and cognition and are tightly interconnected. The mechanisms in which the human body responses lead to weigh gain are discussed in the following subsections.

Physiological triggers

Stress activates multiple physiological systems in the human body of which three are conducive to overweight and obesity, which are: hypothalamic-pituitary-adrenal (HPA) axis activation, reward processing and microbiome (Tomiyama 2018).

When an individual perceives stress, HPA axis sends signals to the adrenal glands to secrete the hormone cortisol, which triggers processes that lead to overweight/obesity; i.e., (1) cortisol increases appetite and the motivation to eat (Epel et al. 2001), and (2) cortisol directly promotes fat deposition, particularly in the abdominal region (Björntorp 2001; Shibli-Rahhal, Van Beek and Schlechte 2006). Abdominal obesity is a toxic form of fat deposition that contributes to poor metabolic (insulin resistance) and cardiovascular health (Després, Lemieux and Prud'homme 2001).

Stress independently triggers the release of dopamine, which enhances the desire for seeking and eating foods that are high in sugar, fat and calories (Pruessner et al. 2004, Wand et al. 2007). These palatable foods provide temporary relief/comfort from stressful states, and therefore consuming them becomes entrenched as a reward-driven habit and addiction (Dallman 2010; Avena 2010).

Microbes in the gastrointestinal tract (i.e. gut microbiome) are responsive to psychological stress whereby: (1) they could affect weight gain by increasing stress-related activations of HPA axis (Tilders et al. 1994); (2) they can influence eating behaviour (taste and appetite) (Duca et al. 2012); and (3) they also directly influence body weight (Turnbaugh et al. 2009).

Behaviour

Chronic stress negatively affects healthy behaviour patterns such as eating, sleep, physical activity and alcohol consumption, which contribute to weight gain. Moreover, there are interplays among these behaviour patterns, which further reinforce weight gain.

Tomiyama (2018) argued that stress induces overeating and consumption of foods that are high in sugar, fat and calories (hyper-palatable). Wardle et al. (2000) experimented this situation with work stress in that they found that employees had a higher intake of saturated fat and sugar-rich food during high work overload

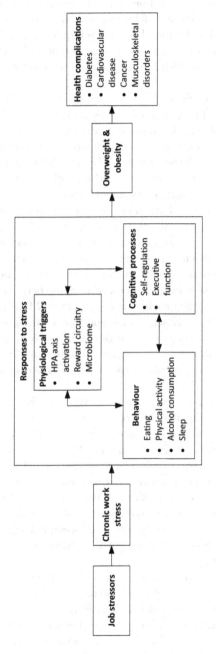

Figure 5.1 Work stress to obesity
Source: Modified from Tomiyama 2018 and Solovieva et al. 2013

periods. Yau and Potenza (2013) argued that highly palatable, energy-dense foods may be addictive, in ways similar to drugs of abuse, and stress is an important facilitator of the development of addiction. This suggests that chronic stress can promote addiction to and overeating of hyper-palatable foods. When one consumes extra calories from food and drinks than what is required for daily living, the body stores the excessive calories. Continued overconsumption leaves a large amount of stored calories in the body, which then translates into abnormal or excessive fat accumulation over time.

Extant literature in public health concludes an inverse bi-directional relationship between stress and physical activity or exercise. Great focus is placed on the antidepressant effects of exercise or physical activity so much so that regular exercise is considered a significant intervention for stress reduction and for improving wellbeing. However, Stults-Kolehmainen and Sinha (2014), after an extensive systematic review of 168 studies that examined the influence of stress on physical activity, argued that the number of people who are engaged in regular physical activities in the event of stressful situations is less than those who become less active. They further concluded that in the majority of cases, psychological stress predicts less physical activity or exercise and/or more sedentary behaviour. Tomiyama (2018) concurred that psychological stress could disrupt activity patterns either by decreasing physical activity and exercise or increasing sedentary behaviour. Longitudinal studies provide evidence for a relationship between higher perceived stress and lower leisure-time activities among women (Mouchacca, Abbott and Ball. 2013). Similarly, Stults-Kolehmainen and Sinha (2014) discovered an association between greater stress and less physical activities regardless of the gender. A lack of physical activity combined with the consumption of excessive calories as explained in the preceding paragraph leads to a higher likelihood of overweight/obesity.

Stress is a well-known disrupter of sleep (Åkerstedt, Kecklund and Axelsson 2007). Shorter sleep duration than the required, which is 7 to 9 hours for adults, has been found to be independently associated with and predictive of overweight and higher likelihood of obesity (Ogilvie and Patel 2017; Patel and Hu 2008). There are three proven mechanisms in which shorter sleep is tied to overweight, which are: (1) shorter sleep reduces one's energy expenditure through reduced thermogenesis – the dissipation of energy through the generation of heat (Shaw 2005); (2) it causes fatigue that contributes to reduced physical activity and increased sedentary behaviour, thus reduced body energy/calorie use (Dinges et al. 1997); and (3) shorter sleep makes people hungrier, particularly for high carbohydrate and fat foods (Spiegel et al. 2004).

Bressert (2018) suggested that many consume alcohol to cope with daily stress from aspects such as job, marital discord and financial challenges, but people with excessive or chronic stress often drink excessively. Traversy and Chaput (2015) found that heavy drinking is consistently related to weight gain. Yeomans (2010) summarised the mechanisms in which alcohol consumption influences weight gain that: (1) 1 gram of alcohol provides 7.1kcal (29kJ) of energy and consuming alcohol with meal increases the energy density of the meal; (2) alcohol intake can increase appetite, leading to increased food intake; and (3) alcohol hinders fat burning, suggesting frequent alcohol intake may result in spare body fat. Moreover, alcohol consumed before bedtime negatively affects sleep which is a contributor to weight gain as elucidated in the preceding paragraph. Roehrs and Roth (2001) reinforced with biochemical explanations that alcohol has extensive effects on sleep quantity and quality and subsequent levels of daytime sleepiness.

Cognitive processes

Heatherton (2011) maintained that self-regulation is essential for controlling one's behaviour related to eating and physical exercise/exercise to prevent obesity. However, Tomiyama (2018) argued that psychological stress interferes with cognitive processes such as executive function and self-regulation, and thus can lead to overweight and obesity. Furthermore, Raio et al. (2013) claimed that psychological stress can prevent cognitive emotion regulations too, thus making individuals even more susceptible to emotional processes that can trigger unhealthy eating.

Effects of individual characteristics

Whilst there is ample evidence to support a direct aetiological pathway from work stress to obesity, there is another set of evidence that places an importance on the role of individual characteristics in the stress–obesity pathway. These may be considered covariates and are summarised as follows:

- Kivimäki et al. (2015) argued that the association between job strain and body weight is inconsistent. Job strain causes mental health problems, which in turn increase or decrease appetite, leading to weight gain in some and weight loss in others. They further claimed that individual differences (i.e. gender and original body weight) play a role in response patterns. On the other hand, they do agree that job strain is a risk factor for type 2 diabetes.
- Solovieva et al. (2013) studied the strength of associations between different psychosocial factors at work and obesity. They found that long work hours had the strongest association with obesity among all the job stressors. They further claimed that the associations between psychosocial factors and obesity were statistically more significant among women than men.
- Poulsen et al. (2014) tested the influence of the demographic factors such as gender, age, ethnicity and living condition (alone/partnered) on the causal relationship between work stress and obesity and found that age and ethnicity have a stronger moderating effect on the relationship.
- van der Valk et al. (2018) claimed that stress may play a major role in the development and maintenance of obesity in individuals who have an increased glucocorticoid sensitivity, which is partly genetically determined. Individual responses to stress can also be influenced by genetic factors (Solovieva et al. 2013).

In summary, chronic work stress activates physiological changes, which promote fat deposition, and metabolic health in their own right. Chronic work stress may also lead to unhealthy eating, physical inactivity, sleep deprivation and alcoholism, and these four factors form a complex interplay among themselves. Moreover, the interplay is further reinforced by the negative physiological and cognitive triggers caused by stress. These collectively contribute to overweight and obesity. The gender, age, original weight and ethnicity of an individual can be covariates in the causal pathway. Moreover, overweight/obesity elevates the vulnerability to type 2 diabetes, cardiovascular disorders, musculoskeletal disorders and certain types of cancer.

Research method

The literature review in the previous section provides a generic theoretical background and propositions around the subject matter. The research discussed in this chapter tests their applicability in the context of professionals working in the construction industry whereby it investigates the following:

- What is the prevalence of work stress induced weight gains among construction professionals?
- What are the most significant job stressors that cause weight gain?
- How do individual characteristics influence work stress induced weight gain?
- How does work stress induced weight gain affect job outcomes?
- How do individual stress coping styles affect weight gain?
- How do work stress induced weight gains affect physical and mental health?

Data

Data required for this study were collected through an online questionnaire survey in the Australian construction industry. Details of the questionnaire, survey administration and respondents were discussed in the previous chapters and therefore are not repeated here, but the data related to this chapter are summarised in Table 5.1. Moreover, a copy of the survey instrument can be found in the Appendix.

A total of 310 construction professionals participated in the survey, but only 247 responses were complete and could be used for analysis. This was above the minimum required number of 241 for a survey that collects responses on a 4-point Likert scale with a 95% confidence level, as per Park and Jung (2009). Refer to Table 1.3 in Chapter 1 for socio-demographic details of the survey respondents. Except for the socio-demographic details of the respondents, the respondents were requested to respond to most questions on a 4-point Likert scale, which were coded numerically in the following manner to facilitate quantitative analyses:

- Scale 1: never = 0, sometimes = 1, often = 2, always = 3.
- Scale 2: not satisfied = 0, somewhat satisfied = 1, satisfied = 2, very satisfied = 3.
- Scale 3: never = 0, once or twice = 1, monthly = 2, weekly = 3.
- Scale 4: not at all = 0, several days = 1, more than half the days = 2, nearly every day = 3.

Analysis techniques

Multiple analysis techniques were used to answer the research questions as outlined in the following:

- The prevalence of work stress induced weight gain was assessed using descriptive statistics, along with inferential techniques such as one-sample t-tests for population.
- Kruskal-Wallis H tests were performed to investigate how the differences in individual characteristics influence weight gain.
- Cluster analysis was performed to investigate the relationship of weight gain with job stressors, work stress, stress coping methods, mental disorders and job outcomes. Cluster analysis helps grouping of data based on their characteristics and enables the identification of most significant data characteristics that are pertinent to an outcome. The merits of this analytics technique were explained in Chapter 3.
- Pearson bi-variate correlation analysis was conducted to examine the association between weight gain and physical and mental health issues among construction professionals.

Construction professionals and work stress induced weight gain

The findings of the analyses geared towards addressing the research questions outlined earlier are elucidated in this section under suitable subheadings.

Prevalence of work stress induced weight gain

Descriptive statistical analyses were conducted to understand the prevalence level of work stress induced weight gain and their severity spreads among construction industry professionals who responded to the survey. Participants' responses to the following two questions were studied:

A) In the past 6 months how often were you bothered by/treated for weight gain/obesity?
   - Never
   - Once or twice
   - Monthly
   - Weekly

B) Do you believe that job stress may have caused this illness?
   - No
   - Yes

Table 5.1 Data related to work stress induced weight gain

Section	Response options

Respondent's background

1. Gender (male, female or other)
2. Age (≤20, 21–30, 31–40, 41–50, 51–60 or >60)
3. Marital status (married/de-facto, single or divorced/separated/widowed)
4. Organisation type (property development, PM, architecture, engineering, QS, builder, subcontractor, FM or other)
5. Organisation size (measured by # of full-time employees) (≤4, 5–19, 20–199 or ≥200)
6. Job title (text responses were received but categorised as junior professional, mid-career professional, senior professional or executive)
7. Experience (<1 year, 1–5 years, 6–10 years or >10 years)
8. Nature of employment (permanent, fixed-term contract or casual)
9. Hours worked weekly (<20, 20–30, 30–40, 40–50 or >50)
10. Workplace environment (site or office)
11. Income (<$40k, $40–60k, $60–80k, $80–100k, $100–120k, $120–150k or >$150k)

Job stressors

In the past 6 months at work how often did you experience: Measured using the scale of:

1. Poor/dangerous work environment   • Never
2. Excessive workload   • Sometimes
3. Unpredictable work hours   • Often
4. Time pressure   • Always
5. Job autonomy
6. Job appropriateness
7. Flexibility
8. Supportive feedback
9. Line manager support
10. Co-worker support
11. Harassment
12. Bullying
13. Discrimination
14. Role ambiguity
15. Adequate job resources
16. Staff consultation
17. Sufficient remuneration
18. Reward
19. Job security
20. Career prospect

Work–private life conflict

In the past 6 months how often did you experience: Measured using the scale of:

1. Lack of energy for private life   • Never
2. Lack of time for private life   • Sometimes
3. Family complained about too much work   • Often
4. Other personal life stressors   • Always

Chronic job stress

In the past 4 weeks how often did you experience: Measured using the scale of:

1. Poor sleep   • Never
2. Restlessness   • Sometimes
3. Irritability   • Often
4. Tensed   • Always
5. Nervousness

Table 5.1 Cont.

Section	Response options
Stress coping methods	
In the past 4 weeks how often did you engage in the following stress coping methods:	Measured using the scale of:
1. Problem-solving	• Not at all
2. Positive reappraisal	• Several days
3. Seeking support	• More than half the days
4. Relaxation	• Nearly everyday
5. Physical activity	
6. Leisure and humour	
7. Eating balanced diet	
8. Adequate sleep	
9. Isolation	
10. Alcohol/drug use	
11. Smoking	
12. Emotional eating	
13. Criticise/blame others	
14. Compulsive spending	
15. Denial/ignoring as if nothing happened	
16. Releasing tension	
Physical and mental health effects	
A) In the past 6 months how often were you bothered by/ treated for:	Measured using the scale of:
1. High blood pressure	• Never
2. High cholesterol	• Once or twice
3. High blood sugar level	• Monthly
4. Angina	• Weekly
5. Heart muscle weakening	
6. Heart attack	
7. Stroke	
8. Diabetes	
9. Weight gain/obesity	
10. Gastrointestinal disorders	
11. Asthma	
12. Bronchitis	
13. Pneumonia	
14. Eczema	
15. Chronic headache/migraine	
16. Insomnia	
17. Back, neck or shoulder pain	
18. Arthritis	
19. Blurred eye vision	
20. Slow healing	
21. Sexual dysfunction	
22. Reproductive system disorder	
23. Burnout	
24. Anxiety	
25. Depression	
B) Do you believe that your job is the primary cause? (this was asked for each heath problem above)	Dichotomous response –Yes / No
Job outcomes	
In the past 6 months how would you rate your:	Measured using a scale of 1 (low) to 10 (high)
1. Job satisfaction	
2. Job performance	

As illustrated in Figure 5.2, around 47% of the respondents indicated that they suffer from obesity or weight gain, but only 34% of them claimed that it was work induced. Hence, to make further analysis robust, the 13% responses that had indicated 'no' to the question whether it was caused by their job were removed from further considerations. Altogether 43 responses were filtered out, which also included responses with missing values for the two questions listed on page 141. The descriptive analysis was repeated with the filtered data and Figure 5.3 illustrates the results in which both the percentage with obesity and the respondents who indicated that it was work induced are the same. Then, one sample t-test was undertaken to check whether the sample statistics are generalisable to the population. Results are shown in Figure 5.3c. It can therefore be concluded that

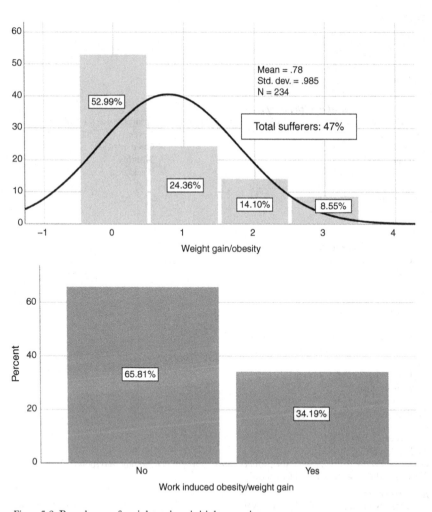

Figure 5.2 Prevalence of weight gain – initial screening

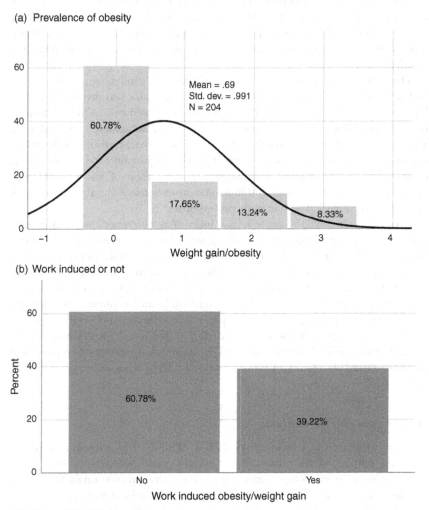

(a) Prevalence of obesity

Mean = .69
Std. dev. = .991
N = 204

60.78%

17.65%

13.24%

8.33%

Weight gain/obesity

(b) Work induced or not

Percent

60.78%

39.22%

No   Yes

Work induced obesity/weight gain

(c) One sample t-test results

One-sample statistics				
	N	Mean	Std. deviation	Std. error mean
Weight gain / Obesity	204	.69	.991	.069

One-sample test						
				Test value = 0.7		
					95% Confidence interval of the difference	
	t	df	Sig. (2-tailed)	Mean difference	Lower	Upper
Weight gain / Obesity	−.127	203	.899	−.009	−.15	.13

Figure 5.3 Prevalence of work induced weight gain

approximately 8% of construction professionals in Australia endure severe work stress induced weight gain and the value changes to around 13% and 18% for moderate and mild severity, respectively. In total, around 39% of construction professionals suffer from work stress induced weight gain in Australia with varying severity levels.

The influence of individual characteristics such as gender, age, marital status and occupation level on work stress induced weight gains was investigated using Kruskal-Wallis H tests. Kruskal-Wallis H test was chosen over ANOVA because the subgroups did not meet the normality and equal subsample size conditions. Table 5.2 presents the test results. Out of the four characteristics, only gender demonstrates an impact on work stress induced weight gain experiences among construction professionals as demonstrated by the p-value of less than .05. The mean rank values further suggest that female professionals suffer more from work stress induced weight gain than male professionals.

Kivimäki et al. (2015) argued that individual differences such as gender and original body weight play a role in stress induced weight gain patterns. Similarly, Solovieva et al. (2013) claimed that the associations between psychosocial factors and obesity were statistically significant more among women than men. Poulsen et al. (2014) found that age and ethnicity have a stronger moderating effect on the relationship. The present study only confirms the influence of gender on the relationship between psychosocial factors and weight gain, and it squarely concurs with Solovieva et al. (2013) that female professionals suffer more. Furthermore, Affenito et al. (2012) claimed that women are represented more than men in overweight statistics globally. The present study concurs with this statistic.

Weight gain cluster analysis

Two-step clustering was conducted on IBM SPSS 26.0 to investigate naturally occurring patterns of the relationship of weight gains with stressors, work stress, stress coping styles and job performance of construction professionals. IBM SPSS has three options for clustering, namely k-means, hierarchical and two-step. Two-step clustering was chosen because it offers the flexibility to process both continuous and nominal/categorical data and it is a combination of non-hierarchical and hierarchical methods. The clustering analysis was performed, involving two successive steps as follows:

- Two-step clustering technique was used to group the cases into n = k clusters by maximising between-cluster differences and minimising within-cluster variances in weight gain and other variables concerned.
- Statistical tests for comparing means of independent samples were used to validate and confirm whether the clusters differed significantly for all variables included in the analyses.

Table 5.2 Impact of individual characteristics on weight gain

Factor		N	Mean Rank	Null hypothesis	Kruskal-Wallis H	Sig.	Decision
Gender	Male	163	97.24	Work stress induced weight gain is the same across different genders of professionals	8.918	**.012**	**Reject null hypothesis**
	Female	38	121.78				
	Other	3	144.17				
Age	Below 20	0	–	Work stress induced weight gain is the same across different age categories of professionals	1.658	.894	Retain null hypothesis
	20 to 30	62	105.52				
	31 to 40	53	97.45				
	41 to 50	49	102.00				
	51 to 60	28	108.14				
	Over 60	11	101.32				
	Unspecified	1	62.50				
Marital status	Married/de-facto	142	98.02	Work stress induced weight gain is the same across professionals with different marital status	6.740	.150	Retain null hypothesis
	Never married	50	109.15				
	Separated	7	128.00				
	Widowed	4	143.75				
	Unspecified	1	62.50				
Occupation level	Junior	49	105.46	Work stress induced weight gain is the same across different occupational levels of professionals	3.796	.434	Retain null hypothesis
	Mid-career	50	109.98				
	Senior	68	95.23				
	Executive	34	99.03				
	Unspecified	3	133.67				

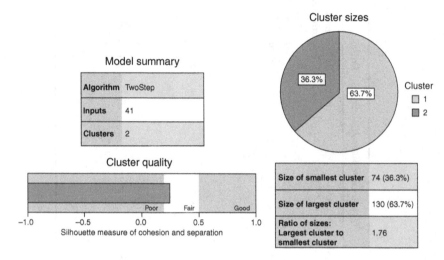

Figure 5.4 Cluster summary

The clustering examined the relationship of weight gain with work stress, job stressors, stress coping habits and job outcomes. The analysis included data gathered on all the 20 stressors, work stress as an aggregation of the five indicators, work–life conflict as a representative cumulative factor of four indicators, all the 16 stress coping methods, job satisfaction and performance levels, and weight gain. The analysis produced two clusters with a ratio of sizes with a value of 1.76, which is smaller than the allowable maximum threshold value of 2.00 (see Figure 5.4). The overall cluster quality was moderately fair and cluster 1 represented 63.7% of the respondents and cluster 2 accounted for 36.3%.

Table 5.3 presents the severity of stressors, work stress, stress coping habits, weight gain and job impact across the clusters. It also depicts the independent sample t-test results that investigated the significance of mean differences of the stressors, work stress, stress coping, weight gain and job impact across the clusters. The p-values yielded for 39 out of 41 variables in the clusters are less than the significant value of .05, suggesting that the two clusters are significantly different and represent two distinct subgroups of construction professionals.

Cluster 2 appears to represent construction professionals whose levels of perceived work stress and weight gain are more than double of those in cluster 1. A close examination of the mean values yielded for the stressors reveal that construction professionals who suffer higher levels of weight gain endure the following stressors at about double the rate of those who are in cluster 1:

- work overload
- time pressure
- lack of support at work
- career stagnation
- work–life conflict.

Table 5.3 Clustering outputs

Variables	Clusters				t-test results	
	Cluster 1		Cluster 2			
	Mean	S	Mean	S	T- stat.	p-value
Weight gain	.66	.920	1.05	1.097	−2.730	.007
Work stress	.8077	.4799	1.8541	.62575	−13.376	.000
Stressors:						
I had to work in poor or dangerous physical work conditions	.12	.321	.62	.696	−7.082	.000
I had excessive workload	1.10	.645	2.09	.762	−9.905	.000
I had unpredictable working hours	1.15	.628	2.12	.721	−10.022	.000
I had excessive time pressures	.96	.791	1.49	.864	−4.405	.000
I had a choice/say in deciding how I do my work	2.08	.778	1.49	.864	5.070	.000
The work I performed was appropriate for my skills and abilities	2.48	.587	2.00	.721	5.208	.000
I had flexibility with my working time	2.22	.726	1.61	.755	5.661	.000
I was given supportive feedback on the work I do	2.05	.697	1.01	.585	10.848	.000
I could rely on my line manager to help me out with a work problem	2.03	.914	1.05	.809	7.641	.000
If work got difficult, my colleagues helped me	2.10	.897	1.32	.878	5.987	.000
I was subject to harassment in the form of unkind/ unwanted words or behaviour at work	2.03	.787	1.19	.753	7.460	.000
I was subject to bullying at work	1.92	.841	1.04	.784	7.383	.000
I was subject to discrimination due to my gender, age or ethnic background	.10	.301	.86	.782	−9.945	.000
I was clear what my duties and responsibilities were	.09	.362	.69	.810	−7.240	.000
I had enough resources to go do my work	.15	.383	.57	.742	−5.253	.000
I was consulted on matters/ changes that affected my job	1.67	.910	1.14	.849	4.128	.000
My salary was sufficient for the work I had to do	1.98	.880	1.19	.788	6.440	.000
I had job security	2.42	.607	1.58	1.007	7.385	.000

(*continued*)

Table 5.3 Cont.

Variables	Clusters					
	Cluster 1		Cluster 2		t-test results	
	Mean	S	Mean	S	T- stat.	p-value
I received reward/ appreciation for the efforts I put into my work	2.13	.730	1.23	.853	7.966	.000
I had career progress opportunities	1.95	.897	.96	.801	7.908	.000
Work–life conflict	.9769	.55897	1.7838	.62390	−9.500	.000
Stress coping methods:						
Problem-solving	.92	.937	1.22	.983	−2.110	.036
Keeping a positive attitude	1.48	1.051	1.41	1.072	.464	.643
Seeking external support	.91	.849	1.36	1.080	−3.344	.001
Relaxation	.66	.859	.70	.856	−.330	.742
Physical activity	1.18	.955	.82	.984	2.563	.011
Engaged in humour, fun and leisure activities	1.49	.856	1.12	.875	2.950	.004
Eating well-balanced meals	1.85	.936	1.51	.969	2.410	.017
Resting and sleeping enough	1.58	.913	.95	.920	4.790	.000
Escape – isolating from others	1.34	.961	1.69	1.072	−2.403	.017
Numbing – consuming alcohol or drugs to forget the stressful situation	.50	.718	1.36	1.130	−6.681	.000
Smoking to get a relief from stress	.18	.590	.49	.910	−2.943	.004
Emotional eating and drinking	.90	.963	1.69	1.097	−5.346	.000
Criticising or blaming others for the situation	.37	.572	1.55	1.036	−10.532	.000
Compulsive spending	.33	.488	.72	.884	−4.014	.000
Ignoring as if nothing happened (denial/ distancing)	.55	.727	1.14	1.064	−4.620	.000
Releasing tension by crying, yelling, throwing things, etc.	.22	.482	.69	.875	−4.992	.000
Job outcomes:						
How would you rate your level of satisfaction with your current job? (1 = low; 10 = high)	7.68	1.337	4.22	1.953	14.972	.000
How would you rate your overall job performance on the days you worked during the past 4 weeks (28 days)? (1 = low; 10 = high)	7.97	1.311	5.80	2.239	8.743	.000

Moreover, they experience role ambiguity and discrimination due to their age, gender or ethnic background at a rate of about eight times higher than that of the professionals in cluster 1.

The examination was further extended to investigate stress coping habits that are prevalent among construction professionals who endure worse work stress and weight gain. It was discernible that professionals in cluster 2 adopt positive coping methods such as problem-solving, keeping a positive attitude, seeking external support, relaxation, physical activity, humour and balanced diet. However, they also adopt the following negative coping habits at a level higher than the positive coping habits. They resort to the following habits at about two to three times the rate of those in cluster 1:

- poor sleep
- alcohol/drug consumption
- consuming comfort food and drinks
- smoking
- compulsive behaviour, particularly spending
- aggressive behaviour such as blaming and releasing tension
- denial/ignoring.

The level of job satisfaction among cluster 2 members is below average (mean value of 4.22 out of 10) and their job performance is only slightly above average (mean value of 5.80 out of 10). In other words, the job outcome is only moderate for the cohort of construction professionals who endure work stress induced weight gain.

Knowledge on work stress induced weight gain is limited, particularly in the construction literature. There is no detailed information about significant stressors that are conducive to weight gain. Solovieva et al. (2013) argued that the strength of associations between different psychosocial factors at work and obesity/weight gain is inconsistent, with long work hours being the strongest predictor. The present study confirms that excessive workload and time pressure, which naturally result in long work hours, are the strongest stressors. The study further finds that lack of support at work, career stagnation and work–life conflict are likewise stronger.

Tomiyama (2018) argued that chronic stress induces addiction to foods that are high in sugar, fat and calories and addictive consumption of such foods can lead to weight gains. The present study confirms that eating comfort foods was rampant among construction professionals who reported work stress induced weight gain. Similarly, Traversy and Chaput (2015) claimed that heavy drinking was consistently related to weight gain. Roehrs and Roth (2001) added that alcohol has extensive effects on sleep quantity and quality. The present study reveals that those who endure stress induced weight gain drink heavily and sleep inadequately.

There is a mix of propositions about the association between smoking and weight gain. There is a general perception that smoking prevents weight gain. This perception was supported by Ghinawi et al. (2016) who claimed that obesity was most prevalent in ex-smokers and least prevalent among current smokers. Similarly, Courtemanche, Tchernis and Ukert (2018) asserted that because nicotine is a metabolic stimulant and appetite suppressant, quitting or reducing smoking could lead to weight gain. The other side of this argument is that smoking could reduce body weight. However, Dale, Mackay and Pell (2015) contradicted this proposition and asserted that the risk of obesity diminished gradually among ex-smokers in proportion to the time since they quit smoking and the risk of obesity increased among current smokers in proportion to the amount smoked. The current study reveals that smoking as a stress coping method is positively associated with stress induced weight gain.

Evidence has been repeatedly established for an association between overweight and emotional behaviour problems such as aggression and withdrawal in children and adolescents. The conclusion was that children and adolescents who are overweight or obese are more physically aggressive than their normal-weight or underweight peers. The proposition here is that physical aggression is a dependant variable and overweight is an independent variable (Tso et al. 2017). Though the present study considered adult professionals as study subjects and they cannot be entirely compared with schooling children and adolescents, it can be argued that there is a relationship between overweight and emotional behaviour problems in humans. The findings of the present study claim that stressed out professionals may adopt aggressive behaviour such as blaming others and releasing tension by yelling or crying as well as withdrawal. There could be a complex interplay among work stress, weight gain, emotional behaviour patterns and mental health as depicted in Figure 5.5. Work stress induces weight gain and emotional behaviour patterns. Weight gain further predicts mental health issues, which reinforces emotional behaviour.

In summary, the cluster analysis reveals complex associations and possibly predictive relationships among job stressors, work stress, stress coping styles and weight gain. Whilst stressors and work stress can predict stress coping behaviour and weight gain in a single direction, weight gain and maladaptive stress coping habits can form a closed feedback loop.

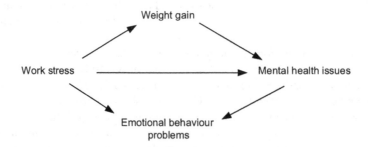

Figure 5.5 Emotional behaviour and weight gain

Association between weight gain and physical and mental diseases among construction professionals

Associations of work stress induced weight gain with other physical and mental diseases among construction professionals were assessed using Pearson correlation analysis. Table 5.4 presents the results. Correlation coefficients below .30 represent weak associations, those between .30 to .70 indicate moderate and those above .70 characterise strong associations (Nardi 2014). Based on this guideline, it is arguable that work stress induced weight gain does not have a strong correlation with any subsequent physical or mental diseases, but there are some moderate and weak associations. Mental health conditions such as depression, burnout, anxiety and insomnia depict the strongest associations with work stress induced weight gain among construction professionals. This is followed by physical health issues such as gastrointestinal disorders, high blood pressure and blurred eye vision. Other health conditions such as cardiovascular disorders and musculoskeletal disorders only showed weak correlations with weight gain in this study.

Table 5.4 Correlations between weight gain and diseases

Health problem	Weight gain	
	Correlation coefficient	Sig. (2-tailed)
Depression	.476**	.000
Burnout	.404**	.000
Insomnia	.374**	.000
Anxiety	.341**	.000
Gastrointestinal disorders	.340**	.000
High blood pressure	.318**	.000
Blurred eye vision	.313**	.000
High cholesterol	.294**	.000
Arthritis	.274**	.000
Angina	.271**	.000
Back, neck or shoulder pain	.263**	.000
Sexual dysfunction	.259**	.000
High blood sugar level	.247**	.000
Heart muscle weakening	.237**	.000
Weakened immune system	.233**	.000
Heart attack	.223**	.001
Eczema	.215**	.001
Migraine or chronic headache	.184**	.005
Bronchitis	.155*	.019
Stroke	.146*	.026
Reproductive system disorders	.132*	.045
Pneumonia	.123	.061
Asthma	.081	.219

** Correlation is significant at the .01 level (2-tailed).
* Correlation is significant at the .05 level (2-tailed).

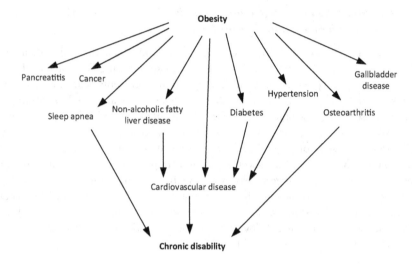

Figure 5.6 Obesity induced diseases
Source: Modified from Pi-Sunyer 2009

The correlations discussed here cannot be concluded as causal relationships. However, evidence from the medical literature supports that these correlations in essence represent causations. Pi-Sunyer (2009) summarised the causal pathway from obesity to other diseases as illustrated in Figure 5.6. Pi-Sunyer (2009) argued that obesity is a significant contributor to increased morbidity and mortality due to cardiovascular disorder, diabetes and cancer. It also contributes to chronic diseases such as osteoarthritis, liver and kidney disease, sleep apnea, and depression. The present study confirms the associations between weight gain and many prevalent diseases with varying strengths. However, construction professionals are more vulnerable to mental health conditions such as depression, burnout, anxiety, insomnia and physical conditions such as vision impairment, gastrointestinal disorders and hypertension due to suffering work stress induced weight gain. Furthermore, complex interconnections are plausible among work stress, weight gain, poor mental health conditions (depression, burnout, anxiety and insomnia) and physical diseases such as vision impairment, gastrointestinal disorders and hypertension. Individuals who are overweight or obese suffer from weight stigma that further worsens their stress. Similarly, any complications caused by being overweight further restrict their physical abilities, worsening mental stress. Overall, a vicious cycle is formed in the stress-overweight pathway.

Conclusion

Overweight and obesity have traditionally been linked to diet and lifestyle. Recently, stress, including work stress, has been found to be a significant contributor as well,

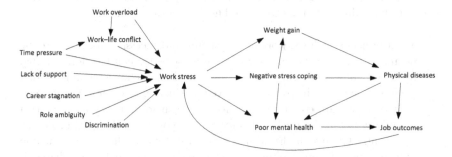

Figure 5.7 Interconnectedness among work stress, overweight and job outcomes

though it is still an underexplored topic in many sectors. This chapter investigated work stress induced weight gain among construction professionals in Australia and reveals several key findings and insights, which are explained here along with Figure 5.7:

•   Around 39% of professionals in the Australian construction industry suffer from work stress induced weight gain. Within this group, 8% suffer severe conditions that require treatment weekly and around 13% and 18% obtain treatment once a month and occasionally, respectively.

•   Female professionals are represented more heavily in the high end of sufferers than are males.

•   The major psychosocial factors that contribute to weight gain among construction professionals are work overload, time pressure, lack of support at work, career stagnation, work–life conflict, role ambiguity and discrimination.

•   Resorting to certain negative habits to manage work stress further reinforces weight gain. The negative stress coping methods are sleep deprivation, alcohol and/or drug use, smoking and consuming comfort foods and drinks.

•   Construction professionals who suffer from work stress induced weight gain have reduced job satisfaction and performance. Their job satisfaction level is only around half of their counterparts and their job performance level is reduced by around one-third.

•   Overweight also contributes to the onset of other health complications. Construction professionals are found to be more vulnerable to vision impairment, gastrointestinal disorders and hypertension due to enduring work stress induced weight gain.

•   The combination of work stress, overweight stigma and the medical complications caused by overweight lead to mental disorders. Both mental disorders and physical restrictions due to diseases undermine job performance. This further adds to work stress level.

Several key implications can be drawn from the study findings for the construction industry, individual professionals and healthcare practitioners:

- Tight project schedules, working long hours and excessive workload are the norms rather than the exception in the present-day construction industry. Moreover, it is still polluted with discrimination. The perception is that having these norms helps with improved production rate. However, it is evident that they are counter-productive, so much so that they not only cost organisations but also the health and wellbeing of the working population of the country. Changes in the norms are required for a productive construction industry and a healthy cohort of construction professionals. The change is not achievable by or the responsibility of a single organisation. Rather a collective effort from different sectors of the construction industry including the government, authorities, clients, institutions, organisations and employees is required.
- Public health policies and interventions that aim to reduce overweight and obesity in the population should focus beyond diet and lifestyle of individuals. They should consider work stress as an equally major risk factor and promote mechanisms and strategies to deploy positive stress coping habits by individuals and primary stress intervention methods by organisations.
- Healthcare specialists generally focus on physical agents for medical conditions. However, this study suggests that they should go beyond that realm and investigate psychosocial factors at work when treating construction professionals for overweight and its subsequent complications such as vision impairment, gastrointestinal disorders and hypertension.
- It is suggested that individual construction professionals adhere to regular exercise to combat both work stress and its effect on weight accumulation. Construction organisations should promote and support their employees to adopt an active lifestyle through programs such as company subsidised gym or sports club memberships. This will pay off through improved productivity and reduced health and safety costs.

References

Affenito, S.H., Franko, D.L., Striegel-Moore, R.H. and Thompson, D. (2012). Behavioral determinants of obesity: research findings and policy implications. *Journal of Obesity*, 2012, article ID 150732. doi:10.1155/2012/150732.

Åkerstedt, T., Kecklund, G. and Axelsson, J. (2007). Impaired sleep after bedtime stress and worries. *Biological Psychology*, 76(3), 170–173.

Australian Institute of Health and Welfare. (2019). Overweight & obesity. Retrieved 2 December, 2019, from www.aihw.gov.au/reports-data/behaviours-risk-factors/overweight-obesity/overview.

Avena, N.M. (2010). The study of food addiction using animal models of binge eating. *Appetite*, 55(3), 734–737.

Björntorp, P. (2001). Do stress reactions cause abdominal obesity and comorbidities? *Obesity Reviews*, 2(2), 73–86.

Bressert, S. (2018). Stress and drinking. Retrieved 3 December, 2019, from https://psychcentral.com/lib/stress-and-drinking/.

Courtemanche, C., Tchernis, R. and Ukert, B. (2018). The effect of smoking on obesity: evidence from a randomized trial. *Journal of Health Economics, 57*(1), 31–44.

Dale, S., Mackay, D.F. and Pell, J.P. (2015). Relationship between smoking and obesity: a cross-sectional study of 499,504 middle-aged adults in the UK general population. *PLoS One, 10*(4), e0123579.

Dallman, M.F. (2010). Stress-induced obesity and the emotional nervous system. *Trends in Endocrinology and Metabolism, 21*, 159–165.

Després, J.P., Lemieux, I. and Prud'homme, D. (2001). Treatment of obesity: need to focus on high risk abdominally obese patients. *BMJ, 322*(7288), 716–720.

Dinges, D.F., Pack, F., Williams, K., Gillen, K.A., Powell, J.W., Ott, G.E., Apstowicz, C. and Pack, A.I. (1997). Cumulative sleepiness, mood disturbance, and psychomotor vigilance performance decrements during a week of sleep restricted to 4–5 hours per night. *Sleep, 20*(4), 267–277.

Duca, F.A., Swartz, T.D., Sakar, Y. and Covasa, M. (2012). Increased oral detection, but decreased intestinal signalling for fats in mice lacking gut microbiota. *PLOS ONE, 7*(6), e39748.

Epel, E.S., Lapidus, R., McEwen, B. and Brownell, K. (2001). Stress may add bite to appetite in women: a laboratory study of stress-induced cortisol and eating behavior. *Psychoneuroendocrinology, 26*(1), 37–49.

Ghinawi, I.A., Bashir, A.I., Alreshidi, Y.Q., Dirweesh, A., Al-Hazimi, A.M., Ahmed, H.G., Kamal, E. and Ahmed, M.H. (2016). Association between obesity and cigarette smoking: a community-based study. *Journal of Endocrinology and Metabolism, 6*(5), 149–153.

Heatherton, T.F. (2011). Neuroscience of self and self-regulation. *Annual Review of Psychology, 62*, 363–390.

Kivimäki, M., Singh-Manoux, A., Nyberg, S., Jokela, M. and Virtanen, M. (2015). Job strain and risk of obesity: systematic review and meta-analysis of cohort studies. *International Journal of Obesity, 39*, 1597–1600.

Mouchacca, J., Abbott, G.R. and Ball, K. (2013). Associations between psychological stress, eating, physical activity, sedentary behaviours and body weight among women: a longitudinal study. *BMC Public Health, 13*, 828. https://doi.org/10.1186/1471-2458-13-828.

Nardi, P.M. (2014). *Doing Survey Research*, 3rd Ed. London: Paradigm Publishers.

Ogilvie, R.P. and Patel, S.R. (2017). The epidemiology of sleep and obesity. *Sleep Health, 3*(5), 383–388.

Park, J. and Jung, M. (2009). A note on determination of sample size for a Likert scale. *Communications of the Korean Statistical Society, 16*(4), 669–673.

Patel, S.R. and Hu, F.B. (2008). Short sleep duration and weight gain: a systematic review. *Obesity, 16*, 643–653.

Pi-Sunyer, X. (2009). The medical risks of obesity. *Postgraduate Medicine, 121*(6), 21–33. doi:10.3810/pgm.2009.11.2074.

Poulsen, K., Cleal, B., Clausen, T. and Anderson, L.L. (2014). Work, diabetes and obesity: a seven year follow-up study among Danish health care workers. *PLOS ONE, 9*(7), e103425.

Pruessner, J.C., Champagne, F., Meaney, M.J. and Dagher, A. (2004). Dopamine release in response to a psychological stress in humans and its relationship to early life maternal care: a positron emission tomography study using [11C]Raclopride. *The Journal of Neuroscience: the official journal of the Society for Neuroscience, 24*(11), 2825–2831.

Raio, C.M., Orederu, T.A., Palazzolo, L., Shurick, A.A. and Phelps, E.A. (2013). Cognitive emotion regulation fails the stress test. *PNAS, 110*(37), 15139–15144.

Ritchie, H. and Roser, M. (2019). Obesity. Retrieved 2 December, 2019, from https:// ourworldindata.org/obesity.

Roehrs, T. and Roth, T. (2001). Sleep, sleepiness and alcohol use. *Alcohol Research & Health*, *25*(2), 101–109.

Shaw, P.J. (2005). Thermoregulatory changes. In C.A. Kushida (Eds.), *Sleep Deprivation: Basic Science, Physiology, and Behavior* (pp319–338). New York: Marcel Dekker.

Shibli-Rahhal, A., Van Beek, M. and Schlechte, J.A. (2006). Cushing's syndrome. *Clinics in Dermatology*, *24*(4), 260–265.

Solovieva, S., Lallukka, T., Virtanen, M. and Viikari-Juntura, E. (2013). Psychosocial factors at work, long work hours and obesity: a systematic review. *Scandinavian Journal of Work, Environment and Health*, *39*(3), 241–258.

Spiegel, K., Tasali, E., Penev, P. and Van Cauter, E. (2004). Brief communication: sleep curtailment in healthy young men is associated with decreased leptin levels, elevated ghrelin levels, and increased hunger and appetite. *Annals of Internal Medicine*, *141*(11), 846–850.

Stults-Kolehmainen, M.A. and Sinha, R. (2014). The effects of stress on physical activity and exercise. *Sports Medicine*, *44*(1), 81–121.

Tilders, F.J.H., DeRuk, R.H., Van Dam, A.M., Vincent, V.A.M., Schotanus, K. and Persoons, J.H.A. (1994). Activation of the hypothalamus-pituitary-adrenal axis by bacterial endotoxins: routes and intermediate signals. *Psychoneuroendocrinology*, *19*, 209–232.

Tomiyama, A.J. (2018). Stress and obesity. *Annual Review of Psychology*, *70*, 703–718.

Traversy, G. and Chaput, J. (2015). Alcohol consumption and obesity: an update. *Current Obesity Report*, *4*, 122–130. DOI:10.1007/s13679-014-0129-4.

Tso, M.K.W., Rowland, B., Toumbourou, J.W. and Guadagno, B.L. (2017). Overweight or obesity associations with physical aggression in children and adolescents: a meta-analysis. *International Journal of Behavioural Development*, *42*(1), 116–131.

Turnbaugh, P.J., Hamady, M., Yatsunenko, T., Cantarel, B.L., Duncan, A., et al. (2009). A core gut microbiome in obese and lean twins. *Nature*, *457*(7228), 480–484.

van der Valk, E.S., Savas, M., and van Rossum, E. (2018). Stress and obesity: are there more susceptible individuals? *Current Obesity Reports*, *7*(2), 193–203. https://doi.org/10.1007/s13679-018-0306-y.

Wand, G.S., Oswald, L.M., McCaul, M.E., Wong, D.F., Johnson, E., et al. (2007). Association of amphetamine induced striatal dopamine release and cortisol responses to psychological stress. *Neuropsychopharmacology*, *32*(11), 2310–2320.

Wardle, J., Steptoe, A., Oliver, G. and Lipsey, Z. (2000). Stress, dietary restraint and food intake. *Journal of Psychosomatic Research*, *48*(2), 195–202.

World Health Organization (WHO). (2018). Obesity and overweight. Retrieved 2 December, 2019, from www.who.int/news-room/fact-sheets/detail/obesity-and-overweight.

Yau, Y.H.C. and Potenza, M.N. (2013). Stress and eating behaviors. *Minerva Endocrinol*, *38*(3), 255–267.

Yeomans, M.R. (2010). Alcohol, appetite and energy balance: is alcohol intake a risk factor for obesity? *Physiology & Behaviour*, *100*(1), 82–89.

6 Work stress induced vision impairment in construction

World Health Organization (2019) estimated that globally at least 2.2 billion people have a vision impairment or blindness. Sabel et al. (2018) considered vision loss irreversible and often progressive, and that affected people experience continuous mental stress, anxiety and depression, resulted from the functional, social and economic restrictions of vision impairment. Eye health conditions such as uncorrected refractive errors, cataract, age-related macula degeneration, glaucoma, diabetic retinopathy, corneal opacity and trachoma are regarded as the immediate medical causes of vision impairment. Recent epidemiological studies have recognised chronic mental stress and associated mental health conditions as significant risk factors for the development and progression of such eye health issues and thereby vision impairment and many other eye problems (Sabel et al. 2018). For instance, Folk (2019) reported a list of eye problems that can be caused by chronic stress, which are: eye movement problems, eye twitching, eye strain, sensitivity to light, tunnel vision, blurred vision and dry eye disease.

Mental stress can originate from various sources such as health conditions, major life changes, financial problems, relationship difficulties, family responsibilities, studies or work. Milenkovic (2019) claimed that workplace stress accounts for a significant portion of the mental health crisis in today's population. It can therefore be deduced that a significant portion of vision-related problems in the working population can be attributed to work stress. Hyon, Yang and Han (2019) demonstrated this empirically in a study involving Korean paramedical workers. Turning to construction, it is conclusive globally that the construction industry is particularly notorious for psychosocial stressors and as a result its professionals endure excessive work stress (Sunindijo and Kamardeen 2017; Bowen et al. 2014; Leung, Chan and Dongyu 2011; Love, Edwards and Irani 2010; Campbell 2006). This suggests that construction professionals are vulnerable to irreversible eye damages and are risking their eye vision. However, this is thus far an underappreciated risk in construction health and safety literature. Hence, this chapter investigates work stress induced vision impairment among construction professionals.

The chapter is laid out in the following manner. First, explanations to different forms of vision impairment are provided. Second, the role of stress and other mental health conditions in mediating vision impairment is explored from an epidemiological perspective. Third, the noise presented by confounding factors in the relationship between stress and vision impairment is outlined. Following that the research method adopted to explore work stress induced vision impairment among construction professionals is detailed. Then, the research and analysis findings are discussed. Finally, conclusions are drawn.

Vision impairment

Vision impairment is a critical health concern that can negatively affect the physical, functional, psychological and social wellbeing and the quality of life of affected individuals. Vision impairment can result from a variety of eye health conditions and Table 6.1 summarises the most prevalent ones along with their risk factors. Vision loss due to some of the conditions are reversible and correctable, some others are irreversible and permanent. The irreversible or permanent vision loss often results from damages to the nerves and retina in the eye. Similarly, some risk factors, such as tobacco, alcohol, diet and regular care, are controllable whilst some others are outside the control of individuals, e.g. age and genetics. Overall, the eye health conditions that cause vision loss and their risk factors are largely attributed to physical and medical circumstances. However, psychological health plays an equally significant role in the health of eyes. Several studies have found associations between different eye conditions that lead to vision loss and stress, anxiety or depression. Some evidence is summarised in the following:

- Lim, Siatkowski and Farris (2015) studied 140 adults and children with functional visual loss and discovered that more than one-third of them were concurrently facing psychosocial problems such as psychological trauma in adulthood or problematic social interactions in childhood
- Yilmaz, Gokler and Unsal (2015) found that individuals with depression, anxiety or stress were more likely to experience dry eye disease
- Sabel et al. (2018) argued that chronic stress and elevated cortisol levels negatively affect the eye and brain and are one of the major causes of visual diseases such as glaucoma and optic neuropathy that can cause irreversible vision loss. Similarly, Diniz-Filho et al. (2016) observed faster visual loss progression in glaucoma with the onset of depression symptoms
- Avetisov et al. (1991; cited in Sabel et al. 2018) claimed a causal role in myopia for stress by studying 762 survivors of the 1988 earthquake in Armenia who had never reported myopia but found 30% of them to have developed it due to life stress resulted by the earthquake
- Hahm et al. (2008) studied patients with retinitis pigmentosa and found that patients with depression had worse vision than those without depression, suggesting depression contributed to faster progression of vision loss.

Sabel et al. (2018) reported that despite the fact that psychological stress is a known risk factor, its causal roles in the development and progression of vision disorders are not widely appreciated.

Table 6.1 Vision impairment

Eye health condition	Definition/characteristic	Risk factors
Age-related macula degeneration	A progressive condition that affects the central part of the retina (macula) at the back of the eye that provides fine vision. It causes irreversible loss of central vision.	Ageing, family history, tobacco consumption.
Cataract	Clouding of the eye's clear lens, reducing the amount of light that passes through it. It causes incorrect focussing of images on the retina, leading to blurred vision. Vision is reversible with a cataract surgery.	Ageing, long-term exposure to sunlight, tobacco, heavy alcohol consumption, diabetes, vascular disease.
Glaucoma	Vision loss or blindness due to damage to the optic nerve. Vision loss caused by glaucoma is not restorable.	High intra-ocular pressure, heredity, extreme short-sightedness, diabetes, hypertension, eye injury, use of steroids.
Diabetic retinopathy	A common diabetes complication that affects the blood vessels of the retina.	Diabetes, high blood pressure, high blood cholesterol, kidney damage.
Refractive errors	Optical defects that prevent light from being properly focussed on the retina, causing long-sightedness, short-sightedness, astigmatism (uneven focus) or presbyopia (problem with near focus).	• For long-sightedness: ageing, genetics. • For short-sightedness: excessive amount of reading, poor metabolism, poor diet, poor light, poor posture, genetic factors. • For astigmatism: genetics, scarring in the eye. • For presbyopia: ageing, long-sightedness, occupation that has near vision demand, ocular disease/trauma, use of drugs such as alcohol, antidepressants and antihistamines, greater exposure to ultraviolet radiation and higher temperature climate.
Trachoma	A chronic conjunctivitis caused by repeated episodes of bacterial infection.	Sub-optimal housing and living conditions.

(continued)

Table 6.1 Cont.

Eye health condition	Definition/characteristic	Risk factors
Eye trauma	Damage caused by a direct blow to the eye. The eye damage can be caused by agents such as impact or blunt force, foreign bodies, chemical injuries or radiation.	Occupations that involve contact with mechanical equipment, chemicals, sources of ultraviolet (welding) or infra-red radiation (furnaces).
Retinitis pigmentosa	Progressive degeneration of the retina due to the inability/reduced ability of the body to supply necessary protein to sustain the retina. It affects night and peripheral vision.	Genetics.

Source: Summarised from Australian Institute of Health and Welfare (2005)

Ocular impact of stress

Scientific literature in the field of psychosomatic ophthalmology, particularly the ones that explore the relationship between stress and vision, is scarce. Sabel et al. (2018) produced a seminal model that explains a circular relationship between stress and eye vision pathology. Figure 6.1 depicts the physiological mechanism in which chronic stress can lead to the onset or worsening of vision loss.

One can experience distress when faced with stressors from any of the sources such as work, life events, financial difficulties or personal circumstances. Similarly, a prognosis of going blind can cause distress and a fearful future as a person with blindness.

The personality trait of an individual plays a key role in stress response. It affects: (1) how an individual appraises or reappraises a stressful event, (2) what coping behaviours are called upon by the individual, and (3) how stress manifests. People with better resilience capabilities manage and cope with the stress well. For example, Benn (1997) postulated two personality traits namely neuroticism and optimism along with five coping habits such as distancing, accepting responsibility, escape-avoidance, effective problem-solving and positive reappraisal. They further argued that optimism and distancing were associated with greater adaptation and coping, whilst neuroticism and escape-avoidance were associated with reduced adaptation to stress.

When the pressure exerted by the stressors and the distress levels experienced exceed the resilience and coping capacities of the individual, this can manifest as psychological symptoms such as stress, burnout, anxiety or depression. Simultaneously, the body will trigger its natural acute stress response, also known

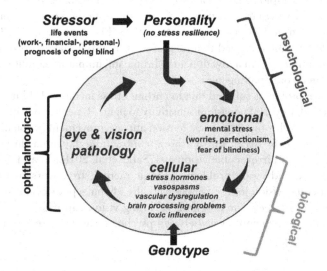

Figure 6.1 The cause–effect relation of stress and vision loss
Source: Sabel et al. 2018

as 'fight or flight response' which subsequently causes the body to secrete stress hormones into the blood stream to prepare the body and mind with the physiological, psychological and emotional changes to deal with the stress.

Many systems, organs and glands in the body undergo stress response changes. Accordingly, changes in the eye include: dilation of pupils to allow more visual information intake, tense and increased blood flow to the eye muscles so that they are more reactive, narrowing of field/peripheral vision so that the focus will be solely on the threat, and a decrease in the blink rate so that important visual information is not missed. Because of these changes, eyes can become dry, eye muscles can feel strained, vision can be more vivid, and one can experience tunnel vision (Folk 2019).

The body recovers to its normal state after the stress has ceased and the stress responses have ended. The body recovers quickly after infrequent stress episodes. However, chronic stress keeps the stress hormone levels elevated, which negatively impact on the eye and brain through different biological mechanisms and aetiological pathways (Sabel et al. 2018). McKlveen et al. (2013) and Lupien et al. (2009) claimed that whilst the release of the hormone cortisol is beneficial during stress for adaptation, the overexposure of the brain to it due to elevated levels resulted from chronic stress can become toxic to neurons and retinal tissues. Na et al. (2010) and Riccadonna et al. (2003) argued that glaucoma is caused by mechanisms such as intraocular pressure elevation, vascular dysregulation and inflammation. Marc and Stan (1990) explained that mental stress elevates intraocular pressure, which reduces the blood flow in the eye, contributing to glaucoma onset and/or rapid progression. Moreover, stress hormones in the vascular system influence vascular tone in and around the optic nerve, impairing vascular autoregulation and thereby ocular blood flow (Flammer et al. 2013). Segerstrom and Miller (2004) argued that mental stress is also a major provocative factor in the immune system activation and chronic inflammatory conditions that contribute to glaucoma pathogenesis.

The resulting eye problems suffered due to chronic stress include: (1) blurred vision, (2) persistent dry eye, (3) persistent sensitivity to light, (4) persistent tunnel vision, (5) eye strain, (6) chronic eye muscle tension and eye movement problems, and (7) eye twitching (Folk 2019). Furthermore, contracting glaucoma due to mental stress may result in irreversible vision loss (Sabel et al. 2018). In addition to causing several eye and vision problems, chronic mental stress worsens the condition and expedites vision loss in people who already have poor eye health conditions. Moreover, the news or prognosis of losing vision can trigger more mental stress, leading to a vicious cycle between psychological stress and losing vision.

Confounding risk factors

Literature suggests several confounding factors that can impose noise on the causal associations between mental stress and vision loss:

- in studying work stress induced dry eye disease among paramedical workers, Hyon, Yang and Han (2019) found an increased prevalence among the female gender and among prolonged users of computers at work
- Lu et al. (2017) and López-Miguel et al. (2014) claimed that such workplace environmental characteristics as low indoor humidity, reduced indoor air flow and exposure to volatile organics make individuals more prone to dry eye disease. Moreover, exposure to ultraviolet or infra-red radiation as well as contacts with chemicals at work or long-term exposure to sunlight were found to be risk factors for eye-trauma-related vision loss (Australian Institute of Health and Welfare 2005)
- when investigating the association between dry eye disease and psychosomatic conditions, Yilmaz, Gokler and Unsal (2015) found that factors such as older age, family history and the use of medications for chronic diseases increase the occurrence of dry eye disease
- Bubella, Bubella and Cillino (2014) claimed that chronic glaucoma was more prevalent among individuals with type A behaviour pattern than type B. Type A is characterised by the presence of an intense drive to achieve goals, persistent desire for recognition and advancement and propensity to accelerate the rate of execution of tasks whilst type B is completely the opposite (Kamardeen and Sunindijo 2017)
- Australian Government, National Health and Medical Research Council (2008) suggested that tobacco use, heavy alcohol consumption, diet and ageing are the most common risk factors for eye diseases and vision loss. Smoking

causes oxidative stress in the eye (Kelly et al. 2005), which subsequently contributes to macula degeneration (Bailey et al. 2004). Alcohol inhibits the absorption of nutrients important to the lens of the eyes (Hiratsuka and Li 2001). Nutrients such as lutein and zeaxanthin, vitamin C, vitamin E and zinc are essential for reducing the risk of certain eye diseases. Inadequate intakes of a balanced diet containing these nutrients is a risk factor for vision loss (American Optometric Association 2020).

In summary, factors such as age, gender, diet, smoking, alcoholism, extensive computer use, physical work and living atmosphere, genetics, regular medication use, and type A behaviour pattern can exert an influence in the relationship between psychological stress and vision loss.

Research method

The preceding sections discussed various risk factors for vision impairment. Figure 6.2 maps out the factors in a concise manner and formulates a conceptual framework for investigating the situation in the context of the construction industry. Accordingly, the following research questions were examined:

- What is the prevalence of work stress induced vision impairment among construction professionals?
- What are the key psychosocial risk factors at work that contribute to vision impairment?
- How do personal and physical workplace characteristics influence the relationship between work stress and vision impairment?
- How do individual stress coping methods influence the relationship between work stress and vision impairment?
- How do other physical and mental health conditions confound work stress induced vision impairment?
- How does vision impairment impact on job outcomes?

Data

Data required for this study were collected through an online questionnaire survey in the Australian construction industry. Details of the questionnaire, survey administration and respondents were discussed in the previous chapters and therefore are not repeated here, but the data related to this chapter are summarised in Table 6.2. Moreover, a copy of the survey instrument can be found in the Appendix. A total of 310 construction professionals participated in the survey, but only 247 responses were complete and could be used for analysis. This was above the minimum required number of 241 for a survey that collects responses on a 4-point Likert scale with a 95% confidence level, as per Park and Jung (2009). Refer to Table 1.3 in Chapter 1 for socio-demographic details of the survey respondents. Except for the socio-demographic details of the respondents, the respondents

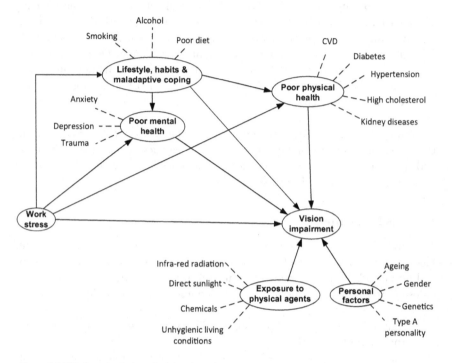

Figure 6.2 Work stress induced vision impairment

were requested to respond to most questions on a 4-point Likert scale, which were coded numerically in the following manner to facilitate quantitative analyses:

- Scale 1: never = 0, sometimes = 1, often = 2, always = 3.
- Scale 2: not satisfied = 0, somewhat satisfied = 1, satisfied = 2, very satisfied = 3.
- Scale 3: never = 0, once or twice = 1, monthly = 2, weekly = 3.
- Scale 4: not at all = 0, several days = 1, more than half the days = 2, nearly every day = 3.

Analysis techniques

Multiple analysis techniques were deployed to answer the research questions as outlined here:

- The prevalence of work stress induced vision impairment was assessed using descriptive statistics, along with inferential techniques such as one-sample t-tests for population.

Table 6.2 Data pertinent to work stress induced vision impairment

Section	Response options

Respondent's background
1. Gender (male, female or other)
2. Age (≤20, 21–30, 31–40, 41–50, 51–60 or >60)
3. Marital status (married/de-facto, single or divorced/separated/widowed)
4. Organisation type (property development, PM, architecture, engineering, QS, builder, subcontractor, FM or other)
5. Organisation size (measured by # of full-time employees) (≤4, 5–19, 20–199 or ≥200)
6. Job title (text responses were received but categorised as junior professional, mid-career professional, senior professional or executive)
7. Experience (<1 year, 1–5 years, 6–10 years or >10 years)
8. Nature of employment (permanent, fixed-term contract or casual)
9. Hours worked weekly (<20, 20–30, 30–40, 40–50 or >50)
10. Workplace environment (site or office)
11. Income (<$40k, $40–60k, $60–80k, $80–100k, $100–120k, $120–150k or >$150k)

Job stressors
In the past 6 months at work how often did you experience:
1. Poor/dangerous work environment
2. Excessive workload
3. Unpredictable work hours
4. Time pressure
5. Job autonomy
6. Job appropriateness
7. Flexibility
8. Supportive feedback
9. Line manager support
10. Co-worker support
11. Harassment
12. Bullying
13. Discrimination
14. Role ambiguity
15. Adequate job resources
16. Staff consultation
17. Sufficient remuneration
18. Reward
19. Job security
20. Career prospect

Measured using the scale of:
• Never
• Sometimes
• Often
• Always

Work–private life conflict
In the past 6 months how often did you experience:
1. Lack of energy for private life
2. Lack of time for private life
3. Family complained about too much work
4. Other personal life stressors

Measured using the scale of:
• Never
• Sometimes
• Often
• Always

Chronic job stress
In the past 4 weeks how often did you experience:
1. Poor sleep
2. Restlessness
3. Irritability
4. Tensed
5. Nervousness

Measured using the scale of:
• Never
• Sometimes
• Often
• Always

(continued)

Table 6.2 Cont.

Section	Response options
Stress coping methods	
In the past 4 weeks how often did you engage in the following stress coping methods:	Measured using the scale of:
1. Problem-solving	• Not at all
2. Positive reappraisal	• Several days
3. Seeking support	• More than half the days
4. Relaxation	• Nearly everyday
5. Physical activity	
6. Leisure and humour	
7. Eating balanced diet	
8. Adequate sleep	
9. Isolation	
10. Alcohol/drug use	
11. Smoking	
12. Emotional eating	
13. Criticise/blame others	
14. Compulsive spending	
15. Denial/ignoring as if nothing happened	
16. Releasing tension	
Physical and mental health effects	
A) In the past 6 months how often were you bothered by/treated for:	Measured using the scale of:
1. High blood pressure	• Never
2. High cholesterol	• Once or twice
3. High blood sugar level	• Monthly
4. Angina	• Weekly
5. Heart muscle weakening	
6. Heart attack	
7. Stroke	
8. Diabetes	
9. Weight gain/obesity	
10. Gastrointestinal disorders	
11. Asthma	
12. Bronchitis	
13. Pneumonia	
14. Eczema	
15. Chronic headache/migraine	
16. Insomnia	
17. Back, neck or shoulder pain	
18. Arthritis	
19. Blurred eye vision	
20. Slow healing	
21. Sexual dysfunction	
22. Reproductive system disorder	
23. Burnout	
24. Anxiety	
25. Depression	
B) Do you believe that your job is the primary cause? (this was asked for each heath problem above)	Dichotomous response –Yes / No
Job outcomes	
In the past 6 months how would you rate your:	Measured using a scale of 1
1. Job satisfaction	(low) to 10 (high)
2. Job performance	

- Kruskal-Wallis H tests were performed to investigate how personal and work environment characteristics influence work stress induced vision impairment.
- Multidimensional scaling technique was applied for identifying job stressors, stress coping habits, mental health conditions and physical health conditions that are pertinent to stress induced vision impairment.
- Structural path analysis was performed to investigate the causal connections linking work stress, coping habits, mental health conditions, physical health conditions, vision impairment and job outcomes.

Construction professionals and work stress induced vision impairment

This section expounds the findings of the data analysis under pertinent sub-headings.

Prevalence of work stress induced vision impairment

Descriptive statistical analyses were performed to examine the prevalence of work stress induced vision impairment among construction industry professionals who responded to the survey. Participants' responses to the following two questions were studied:

A) In the past 6 months how often were you bothered by/treated for blurred eye vision?
- Never
- Once or twice
- Monthly
- Weekly
B) Do you believe that job stress may have caused this illness?
- No
- Yes

An analysis for initial screening revealed that about 31% of the respondents indicated that they suffer from blurred eye vision, but only around 29.5% of them alleged that it is work induced. Hence, the 1.5% of the respondents who indicated 'no' to the question whether it was caused by their job was removed from further considerations to make the analysis robust. Accordingly, altogether 28 responses were filtered out, which also included responses with missing values for the two questions. The descriptive analysis was repeated with the filtered data and Figure 6.3 illustrates the results in which both the percentage with impaired vision and the respondents who indicated that it is work induced are the same. Then, one sample t-test was undertaken to check whether the sample statistics are generalisable to the population. Results are shown in Figure 6.3c. It can therefore be concluded that around 5% of construction professionals in Australia endure

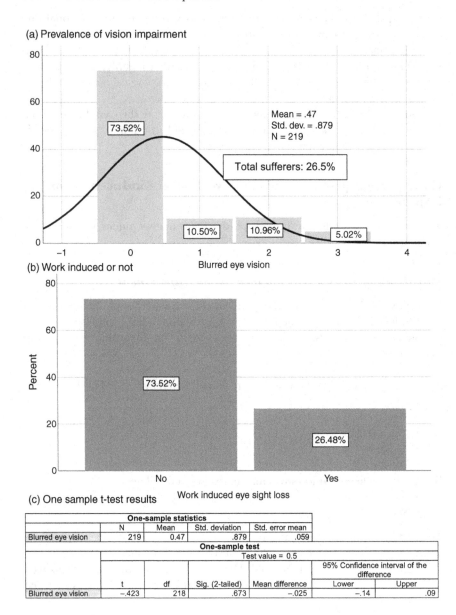

Figure 6.3 Prevalence of work stress induced vision impairment

severe vision impairment due to work stress and the value changes to around 11% for moderate or mild severities. In total, a little over one-fourth of construction professionals suffer from work stress induced vision impairment in Australia with varying severity levels.

Influence of personal and workplace characteristics on work stress induced vision impairment

Kruskal-Wallis H tests were performed to investigate how personal factors such as age, gender and the occupation level as well as the workplace type influence the onset of work stress induced vision impairment. Kruskal-Wallis H test was chosen over ANOVA because the subgroups did not satisfy the equal subsample size condition. Table 6.3 presents the test results.

The gender of construction professionals appears to have a bearing on work stress induced vision impairment as demonstrated by the p-value of less than .05. Moreover, the mean rank values further suggest that female professionals suffer more severely from work stress induced vision impairment than male professionals. The finding aligns with Hyon, Yang and Han (2019) who claimed an increased prevalence of work stress related dry eye disease among the female gender.

Generally, ageing has been linked to vision impairment quite widely in the literature (Australian Institute of Health and Welfare 2005; Yilmaz, Gokler and Unsal 2015). Whilst this may be true for general vision impairment that is mediated by medical conditions, it is not significant in the case of work stress induced vision impairment as suggested by the current research findings.

Existing literature suggests genetics and the type A personality can also have an impact on work stress induced vision impairment. However, the assessment of heredity or genetics is complicated and requires mainstream medical research. Similarly, the personality type of respondents was not gauged in the survey. These limit the analysis of the impact of these factors in the present study.

Literature claims that exposure to low indoor humidity, reduced indoor air flow, volatile organics, ultraviolet or infra-red radiation and direct sunlight at workplace increase the chances of contracting eye health conditions such as dry eye disease and eye trauma, which could eventually lead to vision impairment (Lu et al. 2017; López-Miguel et al. 2014; Australian Institute of Health and Welfare 2005). Construction sites are characterised by all these hazardous agents and therefore it may be expected that site-based professionals would be heavily represented in the statistics for vision impairment. Nonetheless, the present study findings do not suggest such a pattern. It could be because these hazards are physical and Australian construction sites implement appropriate safety measures to control or eliminate their negative impacts on professionals.

In summary, out of the five factors investigated, only the gender difference demonstrated an influence on work stress induced vision impairment among construction professionals.

Identifying predictive stressors, stress coping methods and health conditions

Multidimensional scaling (MDS) approach was applied to identify stressors, stress coping methods and physical and mental health conditions that are closely

Table 6.3 Influence of personal and work environment factors on vision impairment

Factor		N	Mean Rank	Null hypothesis	Kruskal–Wallis H	Sig.	Decision
Gender	Male	183	114.48	Work stress induced vision impairment is the same across different genders of professionals	7.944	.019	**Reject null hypothesis**
	Female	51	137.41				
	Other/unspecified	3	81.50				
Age	Below 20	1	179.00	Work stress induced vision impairment is the same across different ages of professionals	9.779	.082	Retain null hypothesis
	20 to 30	74	118.96				
	31 to 40	57	106.49				
	41 to 50	57	113.16				
	51 to 60	30	138.53				
	Over 60	17	135.76				
Occupation level	Junior	60	107.54	Work stress induced vision impairment is the same across different occupational levels of professionals	4.679	.197	Retain null hypothesis
	Mid-career	56	128.87				
	Senior	77	114.50				
	Executive	38	113.43				
Organisation size	Employees ≤4	22	132.36	Work stress induced vision impairment is the same across professionals from different sizes of organisation	3.022	.388	Retain null hypothesis
	5 to 19	43	120.35				
	20 to199	76	121.81				
	Employees ≥200	95	111.81				
Work environment	Office	197	120.35	Work stress induced vision impairment is the same across different work environments	.670	.413	Retain null hypothesis
	Site	40	112.35				
	Unspecified	0	–				

associated with work stress induced vision impairment. MDS is a data visualisation technique that enables modelling and graphically representing relationships
within a set of variables so that the underlying structure of the relationships can
be understood. This is a widely used approach in many fields such as marketing
(Cooper 1983), tourism (Fenton and Pearce 1988), psychology (Whaley and
Longoria 2008), public health (Kemmler et al. 2002) and engineering (Zhao,
Ukkusuri and Lu 2018) due to its ability to cluster and visually present closely
related objects. However, it is an underutilised analysis technique in the construction management domain despite its merits, but the present study leverages
the capabilities of the technique. Separate episodes of multidimensional scaling
(proxscal) were performed to investigate the relationship of vision impairment
with job stressors and stress coping methods.

The perceptual map shown in Figure 6.4 demonstrates the relationship of
vision impairment with job stressors. The clustering of variables is generally
arbitrary, and the axes have less relevance in terms of clustering. Researchers
are allowed to discover suitable shapes that would well represent a subgroup

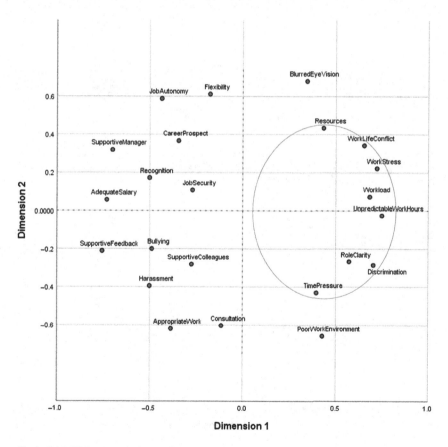

Figure 6.4 MDS perceptual map for job stressors

of variables. The perceptual map shown in the figure clusters job stressors into four quadrants and the stressors in each quadrant represent a different latent construct. For instance, the upper left quadrant appears to represent the characteristics of the job, which may be labelled 'job rewards'. Similarly, the lower left quadrant clusters together stressors that concern 'workplace relationships'. The variable, blurred eye vision, is located in the upper right quadrant along with work stress, suggesting that these two are related factors. Work stress is positioned closer to certain job stressors such as workload, unpredictable work hours, work–life conflict, job resources, role clarity, discrimination and time pressure. These exist both in the lower and upper right quadrants but in similar distances from work stress, as encircled. Hence, it could be deduced that these seven stressors are pertinent to work stress induced vision impairment among construction professionals.

The perceptual map illustrated in Figure 6.5 clusters stress coping methods and identifies the ones that are closely related to vision impairment. The right side of the origin represents positive coping and the left side is negative coping. Coping

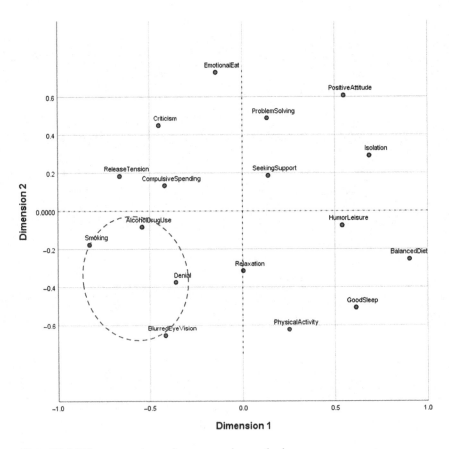

Figure 6.5 MDS perceptual map for stress coping methods

habits in the lower left quadrant are closer to vision impairment. These include smoking, alcohol or drug use and denial/distancing.

The perceptual map shown in Figure 6.6 discovers the mental and physical health conditions that are closely related to vision impairment. The variable, blurred eye vision, is located between mental health conditions such as depression, burnout and anxiety, as well as cardiovascular disorders (CVDs) such as angina, heart muscle weakening, heart attack and stroke. Another cluster comprising such diseases as high blood pressure, high cholesterol, high blood sugar and diabetes is located parallel to CVDs but a bit further away from the location of blurred eye vision. But public health literature claims that these conditions also confound vision impairment.

In summary, the multidimensional scaling findings largely concur with the conceptual framework presented in Figure 6.2, which mapped out the casual paths and predictor variables of work stress induced vision impairment. However, the prediction strengths of these variables are unknown. Knowing them will enable the optimisation of the causal model for targeted prevention.

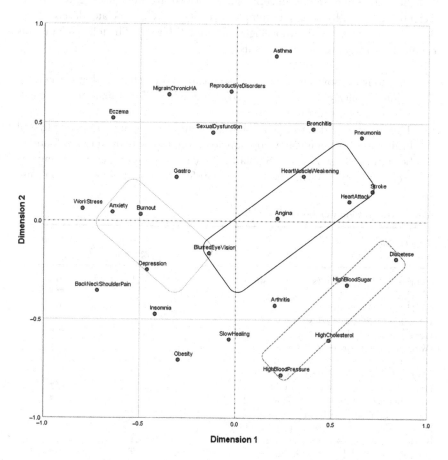

Figure 6.6 MDS perceptual map for mental and physical health

Causal path modelling

Structural path analysis was conducted on IBM AMOS 26 to investigate the strength of predictors of work stress induced vision impairment. Structural path analysis was preferred over other methods because it can simultaneously test a series of cause and effect relationships (Hair et al. 2014).

The conceptual model shown in Figure 6.2 was reproduced on AMOS graphical interface and model testing was performed with the survey data in an iterative manner until a best fitting model for the dataset was achieved. The remodelling process was guided by the modification indices suggested by AMOS and the p-values of the regression weights for prediction paths. Figure 6.7 illustrates the best fitting model, which yielded the following model fit values: CFI = .990, TLI = .979, NFI = .970 and RSMEA = .044. A value close to 1 for CFI, TLI and NFI as well as a value close to 0 for RMSEA suggests a good model fit (refer to Table 4.8 in Chapter 4 for more details about model fit criteria). The final model is slightly different from the conceptual model illustrated in Figure 6.2. Regression weights for the paths, squared multiple correlations (R^2), associated levels of significance (p-values) are shown in Figure 6.7 and Table 6.4. The following insights can be drawn from the analysis results:

- Only four stressors are found to be significant in predicting work stress induced vision impairment, which are work–life conflict, discrimination, unpredictable work hours and work overload.
- The hypothesised causal links between unhealthy coping and poor physical health as well as unhealthy coping and vision impairment were not found to be statistically significant. Similarly, the causal link between vision impairment and job performance drop was not found to be statistically significant.

Table 6.4 Regression weights of direct effects

Direct predictor relationship	Standardised regression weight	p-value
Unpredictable work hours → Work stress	.14	.018
Discrimination → Work stress	.19	***
Workload → Work stress	.12	.05
Work–life conflict à Work stress	.51	***
Work stress → Unhealthy coping	.50	***
Work stress → Poor mental health	.50	***
Work stress → Poor physical health	.16	.009
Work stress → Blurred eye vision	.21	***
Unhealthy coping → Poor mental health	.21	***
Poor physical health → Poor mental health	.27	***
Poor mental health → Blurred eye vision	.22	***
Poor physical health → Blurred eye vision	.26	***
Blurred eye vision → Job satisfaction	−1.16	***
Discrimination → Job performance	−.27	***

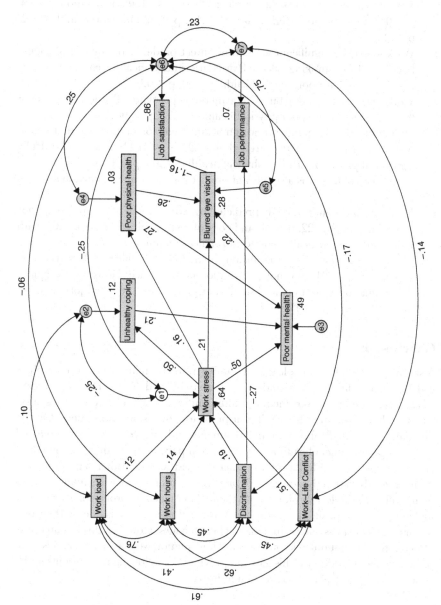

Figure 6.7 Path model of work stress induced vision impairment

However, a new statistically significant causal link between poor physical health and poor mental health is established.

- All four predictors of work stress are statistically significant with varying prediction strengths; i.e. work–life conflict: $\beta = .51$, p <.01, discrimination: $\beta = .19$, p <.01, unpredictable work hours: $\beta = .14$, p <.02 and workload: $\beta = .12$, p <.05.
- Work stress is a significant and strong direct predictor of unhealthy coping habits such as smoking, alcohol/drug use and unhealthy eating $(\beta = .51$, p <.01) as well as poor mental health $(\beta = .50$, p <.02).
- Work stress is a moderate but significant direct predictor of vision impairment $(\beta = .20$, p <.01) and poor physical health $(\beta = .15$, p = .009).
- Unhealthy coping habits are a significant predictor of poor mental health with a moderate predictive strength $(\beta = .21$, p <.01), but not a statistically significant predictor of poor physical health $(\beta = .03$, p = .695).
- Poor physical health is a significant predictor of poor mental health $(\beta = .26$, p <.01).
- Vision impairment is directly predicted by work stress $(\beta = .21$, p <.01), poor mental health $(\beta = .22$, p <.01) and poor physical health $(\beta = .26$, p <.01) with moderate but statistically significant predictive strengths.
- Vision impairment is a significant predictor of reduced job satisfaction $(\beta = -1.16$, p <.01), but not reduced job performance. However, workplace discrimination is a direct and significant predictor of reduced job performance $((\beta = -.27$, p <.01).

Conclusion

A staggering 2.2 billion people globally suffer from vision impairment. Poor physical health conditions have traditionally been blamed for it. However, recent research revealed that poor mental health conditions such as chronic stress, anxiety and depression are also significant predictors of vision impairment. On the one hand, new medical inventions, treatments and interventions are introduced to curtail poor physical health induced vision impairment and the working population is consciously adopting these when needed. On the other hand, they are simultaneously exposed to excessive work stress. This paradoxical situation makes them still vulnerable to vision impairment. Construction professionals are at a highly vulnerable position because the construction industry is one of the worst sectors for work stress and related mental health issues. However, this was an unexplored topic and not much knowledge and information were available on this. The present research addressed this gap and provides the following new insights in the context of the Australian construction industry:

- Around 27% of professionals in the Australian construction industry endure work stress induced vision impairment with varying severity levels; 5%, 11% and 11% of them get treatments for or are bothered by them weekly, monthly and occasionally, respectively.

- The severity of work stress induced vision impairment is higher among female professionals.
- Work–life conflict, work overload, unpredictable work hours and discrimination are the dominant workplace risk factors, which trigger work stress that directly predicts vision impairment in construction professionals.
- Work stress also mediates poor mental health such as burnout, anxiety and depression, and poor physical health such as cardiovascular diseases, diabetes, hypertension and high cholesterol levels among construction professionals. These in turn contribute to vision impairment.
- Certain negative stress coping habits adopted by construction professionals, such as smoking and alcohol/drug consumption, exacerbate work stress induced poor mental health and thereby vision impairment.
- Work stress induced vision impairment significantly reduces job satisfaction among construction professionals though its impact on job performance is not apparent.

Several practical implications might be drawn from these findings:

- The construction industry should consider reforming their work culture and norms. Focus must be placed on reasonable project schedules and project management deadlines as well as family-friendly work hours and work schedules. Better awareness and mechanisms to eradicate discrimination against female professionals should be engrained in the male-dominated construction sector.
- Individual professionals who perceive excessive work stress should avoid resorting to alcohol or tobacco for stress relief. Instead, positive habits such as exercising, recreational activities and healthy diet should be adopted. Construction organisations, professional institutions and unions could promote these positive stress coping strategies regularly and widely.
- Medical professionals who treat construction professionals for vision impairment should not only look into physical health conditions related causes but also work stress and associated mental health conditions as risk factors.

All in all, work stress induced vision impairment can be irreversible. Concerted effort is required from the construction industry bodies, individual professionals, government authorities and the public health sector to curtail it.

References

American Optometric Association. (2020). Diet & nutrition. Retrieved 22 January, 2020, from www.aoa.org/patients-and-public/caring-for-your-vision/diet-and-nutrition.

Australian Government, National Health and Medical Research Council. (2008). Risk factors for eye disease and injury. Retrieved 22 January, 2020, from www1.health. gov.au/internet/main/publishing.nsf/Content/999A85F02A58E9C6CA257C74001 9BE30/$File/risk.pdf.

Australian Institute of Health and Welfare (AIHW). (2005). Vision problems in older Australians. Bulletin no. 27. AIHW Cat. No. AUS 60. Canberra: AIHW.

Bailey, T.A., Kanuga, N., Romero, I.A., Greenwood, J., Luthert, P.J. and Cheetham, M.E. (2004). Oxidative stress affects the junctional integrity of retinal pigment epithelial cells. *Investigative Ophthalmology and Visual Science, 45*(2), 675–684.

Benn, D.T. (1997). The role of personality traits and coping strategies in late-life adaptation to vision loss. Unpublished dissertation, AAI9730084. ETD Collection for Fordham University.

Bowen, P., Edwards, P., Lingard, H. and Cattell, K. (2014). Occupational stress and job demand, control and support factors among construction project consultants. *International Journal of Project Management, 32*(7), 1273–1284.

Bubella, R.M., Bubella, D.M. and Cillino, S. (2014). Type A behaviour pattern: is it a risk factor for open-angle chronic glaucoma? *Journal of Glaucoma, 23*(4), 199–201.

Campbell, F. (2006). *Occupational Stress in the Construction Industry.* Ascot, UK: The Chartered Institute of Building.

Cooper, L.G. (1983). A review of multidimensional scaling in marketing research. *Applied Psychological Measurement, 7*(4), 427–450.

Diniz-Filho, A., Abe, R.Y., Cho, H.J., Baig, S., Gracitelli, C.P. and Medeiros, F.A. (2016). Fast visual field progression is associated with depressive symptoms in patients with glaucoma. *Ophthalmology, 123*(4), 754–759.

Fenton, M. and Pearce, P. (1988). Multidimensional scaling and tourism research. *Annals of Tourism Research, 15*(2), 236–254.

Flammer, J., Konieczka, K., Bruno, R.M., Virdis, A., Flammer, A.J., and Taddei, S. (2013). The eye and the heart. *European Heart Journal, 34*(17), 1270–1278.

Folk, J. (2019). Eye problems, vision anxiety symptoms. Retrieved 13 January, 2020, from www.anxietycentre.com/anxiety-symptoms/eye-vision-problems.shtml.

Hahm, B.J., Shin, Y.W., Shim, E.J., Jeon, H.J., Seo, J.M., Chung, H. and Yu, H.G. (2008). Depression and the vision related quality of life in patients with retinitis pigmentosa. *The British Journal of Ophthalmology, 92*(5), 650–654.

Hair, J.F., Black, W.C., Babin, B.J. and Anderson, R.E. (2014). *Multivariate Data Analysis,* 7th Ed. Harlow: Pearson Education Limited.

Hiratsuka, Y. and Li, G. (2001). Alcohol and eye diseases: a review of epidemiologic studies. *Journal of Studies on Alcohol, 62*(3), 397–402.

Hyon, J.Y., Yang, H.K. and Han, S.B. (2019). Association between dry eye disease and psychological stress among paramedical workers in Korea. *Scientific Reports, 9,* 3783.

Kamardeen, I. and Sunindijo, R.Y. (2017). Personal characteristics moderate work stress in construction professionals. *Journal of Construction Engineering and Management, 143*(10), 04017072.

Kelly, S.P., Thornton, J., Edwards, R., Sahu, A. and Harrison, R. (2005). Smoking and cataract: review of causal association. *Journal of Cataract and Refractive Surgery, 31*(12), 2395–2404.

Kemmler, G., Holzner, B., Kopp, M., Dunser, M., Greil, R., Hahn, E. and Soerner-Unterweher, B. (2002). Multidimensional scaling as a tool for analysing quality of life data. *Quality of Life Research, 11,* 223–233. https://doi.org/10.1023/A:1015207400490.

Leung, M., Chan, Y.S.I. and Dongyu, C. (2011). Structural linear relationships between job stress, burnout, physiological stress, and performance of construction project managers. *Engineering, Construction and Architectural Management, 18*(3), 312–328.

Lim, S.A., Siatkowski, R.M. and Farris, B.K. (2015). Functional visual loss in adults and children patient characteristics, management, and outcomes. *Ophthalmology*, *112*(10), 1821–1828.

López-Miguel, A., Tesón, M., Martín-Montañez, V., Enríquez-de-Salamanca, A., Stern, M.E., Calonge, M. and González-García, M.J. (2014). Dry eye exacerbation in patients exposed to desiccating stress under controlled environmental conditions. *American Journal of Ophthalmology*, *157*(4), 788–798.

Love, P.E.D., Edwards, D.J. and Irani, Z. (2010). Work stress, support and mental health in construction. *Journal of Construction Engineering and Management*, *136*(6), 650–658.

Lu, C., Tsai, M., Muo, C., Kuo, Y., Sung, F. and Wu, C. (2017). Personal, psychosocial and environmental factors related to sick building syndrome in official employees of Taiwan. *International Journal of Environmental Research and Public Health*, *15*(1), 7.

Lupien, S.J., McEwen, B.S., Gunnar, M.R. and Heim, C. (2009). Effects of stress throughout the lifespan on the brain, behaviour and cognition. *Nature Reviews: Neuroscience*, *10*(6), 434–445.

Marc, A. and Stan, C. (1990). Effect of physical and psychological stress on the course of primary open angle glaucoma. *Oftalmologia*, *57*(2), 60–66.

McKlveen, J.M., Myers, B., Flak, J.N., Bundzikova, J., Solomon, M.B., Seroogy, K.B. and Herman, J.P. (2013). Role of prefrontal cortex glucocorticoid receptors in stress and emotion. *Biological Psychiatry*, *74*(9), 672–679.

Milenkovic, M. (2019). 42 worrying workplace stress statistics. Retrieved 16 January, 2020, from www.smallbizgenius.net/by-the-numbers/workplace-stress-statistics/.

Na, K.S., Lee, N.Y., Park, S.H. and Park, C.K. (2010). Autonomic dysfunction in normal tension glaucoma: the short-term heart rate variability analysis. *Journal of Glaucoma*, *19*(6), 377–381.

Park, J. and Jung, M. (2009). A note on determination of sample size for a Likert scale. *Communications of the Korean Statistical Society*, *16*(4), 669–673.

Riccadonna, M., Covi, G., Pancera, P., Presciuttini, B., Babighian, S., Perfetti, S., Bonomi, L. and Lechi, A. (2003). Autonomic system activity and 24-hour blood pressure variations in subjects with normal and high-tension glaucoma. *Journal of Glaucoma*, *12*(2), 156–163.

Sabel, B.A., Wang, J., Cárdenas-Morales, L., Faiq, M. and Heim, C. (2018). Mental stress as consequence and cause of vision loss: the dawn of psychosomatic ophthalmology for preventive and personalized medicine. *The EPMA Journal*, *9*(2), 133–160.

Segerstrom, S.C. and Miller, G.E. (2004). Psychological stress and the human immune system: a meta-analytic study of 30 years of inquiry. *Psychological Bulletin*, *130*(4), 601–630.

Sunindijo, R.Y., and Kamardeen, I. (2017). Works stress is a threat to gender diversity in the construction industry. *Journal of Construction Engineering and Management*, *143*(10), 04017073.

Whaley, A.L. and Longoria, R.A. (2008). Assessing cultural competence readiness in community mental health centers: a multidimensional scaling analysis. *Psychological Services*, *5*(2), 169–183.

World Health Organization. (2019). Blindness and vision impairment. Retrieved 16 January, 2020, from www.who.int/news-room/fact-sheets/detail/blindness-and-visual-impairment.

Yilmaz, U., Gokler, M.E. and Unsal, A. (2015). Dry eye disease and depression-anxiety-stress: a hospital-based case control study in Turkey. *Pakistan Journal of Medical Sciences, 31*(3), 626–631.

Zhao, Y., Ukkusuri, S.V. and Lu, J. (2018). Multidimensional scaling-based data dimension reduction method for application in short-term traffic flow prediction for urban road network. *Journal of Advanced Transportation*, Volume 2018, Article ID 3876841, https://doi.org/10.1155/2018/3876841.

7 Concluding remarks

This chapter concludes the book by summarising the key research findings elaborated in the preceding chapters and their practical implications for construction organisations, construction professionals, government authorities and policy makers, medical practitioners, and the workers' compensation scheme. The chapter further highlights the potentials of the novel analytics methods demonstrated in the book for the benefit of other researchers in construction and other domains. Finally, the chapter outlines possible future research directions to further broaden and deepen the knowledgebase of work stress induced chronic diseases.

Summary of research findings

The construction industry is one of the most vulnerable sectors for excessive work stress for its professionals globally. Public health literature warns that enduring excessive work stress can cause serious chronic diseases. Several studies on work stress in the construction industry have been conducted to date by researchers around the world. However, these investigations were limited to the causes of work stress, stress moderators, stress coping and the effects of stress on psychological health and job performance. Despite its importance, there has been very little research on the relationship between work stress and the development of chronic diseases among construction professionals. This book sets out to discover new knowledge about work stress induced chronic diseases among construction industry professionals by applying analytical methods on data collected in a national survey of construction professionals in Australia. Preliminary findings reported in Chapter 1 reveal that psychological disorders, chronic insomnia, musculoskeletal pains, weight gain/obesity and vision impairment are the predominant health consequences of work stress in the Australian construction industry. Hence, further investigations were conducted into each of these conditions. Key findings are summarised in the following subsections.

Work stress induced psychological disorders

Even though employment is a key determinant of one's quality of life and being unemployed can lead to mental disorders, chronically stressful employments compromise the mental wellbeing of the working population in all sectors and industries. Chapter 2 investigated the prevalence of work stress and work stress induced psychological disorders among construction professionals. The study reveals that:

- Ninety-three percent of construction professionals endure work stress, with 26%, 23%, 28% and 16% suffering low, moderate, high and severe levels of work stress, respectively.
- The primary contributors to work stress in the construction industry are work–life conflict, excessive workload and unpredictable work hours. On the other hand, career progression opportunities, satisfactory salaries, job security and support and consultation culture at work provide a buffer against negative consequences of work stress. Moreover, a significant proportion of professionals who adopt stress coping methods such as thoughtful problem-solving, and leisure and fun activities with socialisation manage work stress well.
- When the workplace lacks buffer factors and/or stressed out employees adopt maladaptive stress coping habits such as aggression, alcohol/drug consumption, emotional eating and drinking, and/or denial/distancing, they develop poor psychological conditions such as burnout, anxiety and depression. Accordingly, 93%, 58% and 47% of stressed out construction professionals reported work stress induced burnout, anxiety and depression experiences, respectively.
- Among them around 15% suffer from severe burnout, anxiety or depression. Moreover, female professionals reported more severe anxiety and depression than their counterpart.
- The implementation of stress management interventions in construction organisations is limited so much so that only large organisations that have employees over 200 adopt secondary and tertiary level stress interventions. Employees of such organisations seem to experience lower work stress, burnout, anxiety and depression as well as higher job satisfaction.

In summary, chronic work stress experience is higher among construction professionals compared to the rate for all employees in Australia, which was estimated to be 75% by Phillip (2019). Moreover, it is evident that burnout is suffered by almost all construction professionals in Australia who endure chronic work stress, but only around half of them experience anxiety or depression symptoms. Nonetheless, the prevalence of mental disorders, particularly anxiety and depression, among construction professionals is much worse than the overall rate of around 20% for Australians, as reported by the Parliament of Australia (2019).

Work stress induced chronic insomnia

Having a good night's sleep is an essential need for good physical health, mental wellbeing and brain functioning for human beings. However, the quality and quantity of sleep is reported to be declining constantly in the working population due to poor psychosocial conditions at work. Chapter 3 studied chronic insomnia due to work stress among construction professionals in Australia and discovered the following:

- About 40% of construction professionals in Australia suffer from moderate to severe chronic insomnia due to work stress, which is more than double the rate of the general population in Australia and other western countries. Moreover, insomnia increases with age and it is more prevalent and severe among female professionals and professionals who belong to micro sized organisations in Australia (i.e. organisations with four or less employees).
- The continued existence of work factors such as excessive workload, unpredictable work hours, work–life conflict, lack of support and resources, and career insecurity and stagnation in the Australian construction industry appear to trigger chronic insomnia, which in turn reduces job satisfaction and performance of construction professionals. The job satisfaction and performance level of affected professionals are lesser by around 40% and 20%, respectively, than the others.
- Construction professionals who suffer from chronic insomnia are more vulnerable to psychiatric conditions such as anxiety, burnout and depression.
- Chronic insomnia is highly correlated with the co-existence of certain poor physical health conditions among construction professionals, which are rapid vision loss, gastrointestinal disorders, weight gain/obesity, musculoskeletal and joint pains, and hypertension.
- Interplays of causal relationships are evident among chronic insomnia, mental disorders and physical ill-health, with one affecting the other bi-directionally.
- Maladaptive stress coping methods such as alcohol and/or drug use, emotional/unhealthy eating and drinking and sedentary lifestyle, which are resorted to by construction professionals, appear to fuel the vicious interplay of causal relationships.

In brief, around 40% of construction professionals who endure chronic work stress suffer from moderate to severe chronic insomnia, which is impacting on their physical health, mental wellbeing and job outcomes. Some of the health impacts are irreversible.

Work stress induced musculoskeletal disorders

Work-related musculoskeletal disorders (WMSDs) are the most prevalent health issue among the working population, and account for 40% of work-related health costs globally. WMSDs have traditionally been believed to be caused by physical force or ergonomic issues at work and therefore were largely attributed to blue-collar operatives, who are generally involved in physically strenuous activities. Nonetheless, recent epidemiological evidence claims that work stress is equally a causal factor, and thus white-collar professionals are likewise susceptible to WMSDs. Chapter 4 explored WMSDs among professionals working in the Australian construction industry, which is one of the worst sectors for work stress.

Among all conditions, back, neck or shoulder pain was discovered to be the dominant WMSD among construction professionals. Forty-five percent of construction professionals in Australia suffer from work stress induced back, neck or shoulder pain and one-third of the 45% receive treatment as frequently as weekly. Moreover, female professionals suffer more severely and receive treatment more frequently than males. Back, neck or shoulder pain among them is caused by a combination of poor psychosocial factors at work and poor stress coping methods adopted by individual professionals. Work–life conflict, excessive workload, unpredictable work hours and excessive time pressure are the key triggers of work stress induced back, neck or shoulder pain among construction professionals. Resorting to stress coping methods such as emotional eating and drinking, alcohol or drug consumption, and aggressive reactions to stress like blaming others and/or releasing tension further aggravates the pain. Surprisingly, job performance and job satisfaction levels of construction professionals were not found to be heavily influenced by their experiences of work stress induced back, neck or shoulder pain.

Work stress induced weight gain

Statistics show that a little over half of the adult population are overweight in the world today. Traditionally, the cause of this was limited to personal factors. Body fat accumulation due to an imbalance between calories consumed and spent, which results from a combination of an increased consumption of calorie-dense food and a sedentary lifestyle, was largely blamed. Hence, overweight or obesity was never regarded as a work health and safety issue. Nevertheless, recent research argues that work stress is a significant risk factor for overweight or obesity in the working population. Chapter 5 investigated work stress induced weight gain among construction professionals in Australia and found that:

- Around 39% of construction professionals in Australia reported work stress induced weight gain, with 8% claiming severe conditions that require treatment weekly, 13% receiving treatment once a month and the remaining 18% receiving occasional treatment. Moreover, female professionals are represented more heavily in the high end of sufferers than are males.
- Seven work related conditions have been found to be the risk factors for this. These are work overload, time pressure, lack of support at work, career stagnation, work–life conflict, role ambiguity and workplace discrimination.

- In addition, seven individual behaviours and stress management habits have been found to be risk factors, which are poor sleep, alcohol/drug consumption, consuming comfort food and drinks, smoking, compulsive behaviour (particularly spending), aggressive behaviour (such as blaming others and/or releasing tension) and denial/ignoring. Whilst the first four of these factors can be directly associated with body fat, the latter three are related to emotional behaviour, which triggers a chemistry in the body that causes weight gain.
- Weight gain develops complicated relationships with physical and mental health. Among construction professionals, work stress induced weight gain demonstrated the strong associations with depression, burnout, anxiety and insomnia, as well as moderate relationships with gastrointestinal disorders, high blood pressure and blurred eye vision.
- Because of the combined and complicated psychological and physiological consequences of weight gain, the job outcome is only moderate for those construction professionals.
- Their level of job satisfaction is around 45% lower and job performance is around 30% lower than other construction professionals.

All in all, work stress induced weight gain is prevalent among around 40% of construction professionals in Australia, whose job outcomes are significantly lower than that of the remaining 60%. Moreover, their mental wellbeing and certain physical health conditions are being affected faster.

Work stress induced vision impairment

World Health Organization asserted that over 2.2 billion people have a vision impairment globally. Recent epidemiological research claimed that chronic mental stress and associated mental health conditions are significant risk factors for the development and progression of vision impairment. Although mental stress can originate from a range of sources for an individual, work stress accounts for a significant portion of the mental health crisis in today's population. Chapter 6 studied work stress induced vision impairment among construction professionals in Australia.

Almost 27% of construction professionals in Australia endure work stress induced vision impairment for which 5% of them receive treatment weekly, another 11% monthly and the remaining 11% occasionally. Moreover, female professionals suffer more severely from work stress induced vision impairment than their counterpart. The vision impairment is the outcome of complex relationships among poor mental health, poor physical health and maladaptive lifestyle, which are triggered by chronic work stress that is in turn caused by four dominant stressors at work viz work–life conflict, work overload, unpredictable work hours and discrimination. Work stress mediates poor psychological conditions such as anxiety and/or depression as well as poor physical health conditions such as cardiovascular disorders, diabetes, hypertension and high cholesterol levels among construction professionals. These subsequently deteriorate eye health and vision.

Work stress also mediates a negative lifestyle characterised by smoking and/ or alcohol/drug consumption in certain professionals, which further reinforces the decline of mental health and thereby eye vision. Work stress induced vision impairment among construction professionals in Australia appears to diminish their job satisfaction strongly.

Opposite patterns

The preceding sections summarised the causes and risk factors for work stress induced chronic diseases. The research also analysed the other professionals who were not affected by these chronic diseases and their work conditions. The following patterns were discernible:

- Factors such as supportive work environment, job security, career progression opportunities and satisfactory salary counteract the adverse effects of stressors. However, when the former factors are also not favourable to construction professionals, work stress is perceived and thereby leads to chronic diseases.
- Construction professionals who encountered stressors but adopted strategies such as thoughtful problem-solving, leisure and fun activities with socialisation and physical exercise/activities managed the stress well and subdued the negative consequences on their mental and physical health.
- Construction professionals who simultaneously deployed negative coping methods such as blaming, distancing and alcohol/drug consumption alongside active problem-solving (positive coping) still experienced moderately high mental strains and their consequences.
- Those professionals who habitually resort to negative coping methods are vulnerable to mental and physical effects even when their actual work stress is low to moderate.

Practical implications

The findings discussed in this book have many practical implications for various stakeholders, namely: the construction industry, construction professionals, government authorities and policy makers, workers' compensation scheme and healthcare/medical professionals.

The construction industry

The construction industry appears to be largely characterised by work overload and time pressure, causing increased work–life conflicts for construction professionals and thereby shaking the stability of their families, which is the basic fabric of a well-functioning society. Whilst there may be a belief that working long and hard can increase the productivity and business return, the construction industry should realise that these are in fact counterproductive and diminishing the physical and mental ability of the talent base of the industry. The following practical measures should be considered for the sustainable development and resilience of the construction industry:

- Realistic project durations should be adhered to in projects. Project durations should not be solely driven by the client's requirement, but the practicality of building a project without compromising the workforce and their families. Models for deciding optimal project durations should be followed and these models should not only factor in project cost but also other project specific constraints.
- The construction industry should be committed to adopting strict work hours and reasonable workload and avoid subtly expecting the workforce to work long hours to meet constant deadlines. A family-friendly work culture should be ingrained in the construction industry. Flexible working arrangements should be promoted heavily and adopted faithfully in organisations of all sizes and types. It is also recommended that weekend and public holidays are strictly declared as non-working days.
- Tailored policies, work arrangements and career pathways should be established to support female construction professionals at all levels of career to both curtail excessive work stress confronting them and to increase female representations in the construction sector without compromising family lives.
- The implementation of the three-tier stress intervention framework should be promoted in the construction industry widely and consistently to nurture a psychosocially sustainable and resilient construction industry that can help build the infrastructure required for the country's economic growth without compromising the social stability. Organisations of all types and sizes in the construction industry should realise their moral obligation and subscribe to a complete implementation of the stress interventions framework faithfully.

Construction professionals

It is quite normal for individuals to turn to quick fixes when confronted with stressors at work. However, resilience should be exercised, and rational options should be adopted to deal with them. It is crucial to internalise that taking quick fixes and shortcuts may provide a short-term solution but mighty destroy the concerned individual's physical and psychological health as well as the family life. The following work habits and lifestyles are encouraged to be adhered to by construction professionals constantly:

- Poor psychosocial issues, stressors and problems at work should be discussed and resolved through respectful open communications and consultations with colleagues and supervisors. Keeping them to oneself is unhealthy and counterproductive.

- The importance of seeking support at the workplace should not be overlooked. This should be done in a manner that is positive for all parties involved at work to reap the best outcome.
- When challenged by mental distress, it is critical that construction professionals do not have self-perceived stigma about their condition, but seek external support from relevant organisations/counsellors to address work stress and its negative impacts on their physical and mental health as well as on the life.
- In all circumstances, construction professionals should maintain a healthy life-style characterised by regular physical exercise, balanced diet, regular leisure activities and adequate relaxation and sleep.
- At all times, shortcut measures such as emotional eating/drinking, smoking, alcohol/drug intake and aggressive responses should be avoided as they can damage the physical and mental health irreversibly though they may seem to provide a quick relief for work stress.

Workers' compensation scheme

Compensation for work-related illnesses is a challenging aspect for construction professionals as they must prove occupational triggers. Similarly, work stress is not compensable in the current workers' compensation scheme unless it leads to reportable/diagnosable psychological disorders. This book established the evidence for the physical and mental health consequences of work stress in the construction industry that can support genuine compensation claims from construction professionals. In the same vein, workers' compensation insurance providers, in addition to conventional physical hazards, may consider assessing the psychosocial risk factors of workplaces to determine appropriate insurance premiums. This will not only minimise their risk exposure but also encourage construction organisations to implement the three-tier stress intervention framework.

Healthcare/medical professionals

Healthcare/medical professionals, when diagnosing construction professionals for chronic diseases such as musculoskeletal disorders, obesity/overweight, diabetes and vision loss, often analyse physical and lifestyle factors. Whilst these are important considerations, the role played by work stress in causing and/or worsening these conditions should not be overlooked. Due psychological diagnoses should be incorporated into the existing model of patient diagnosis and treatment for the previously mentioned chronic diseases, particularly for construction professionals.

Since there is a tendency for patients to be more concerned about physical health issues and their consequences on their quality of life, medical professionals could encourage/reinforce the importance of adaptive lifestyle and habits such as regular exercise, balanced diet and adequate rest as facilitators of good physical health. This will not only help reduce the negative psychological impacts of work stress but also improve physical health simultaneously.

Government authorities and policy makers

Micro and small sized organisations account for a significant portion of the construction industry in any country. They include both builders, subcontractors and consultants who supply services to larger organisations. Despite their size, smooth operations of these organisations are therefore indispensable for the industry and the overall economy. Often these organisations are sole-traders or small partnerships who constantly strive to maintain a decent cashflow, workload and attend to other business matters in addition to personally undertaking project execution. Hence, the owners or employees of these organisations are at high risk of chronic work stress and its negative consequences on their mental and physical health. Supporting this sector of the industry is crucial. It is therefore suggested that policy makers at the federal, state and local government levels establish a support scheme for such businesses and the scheme may comprise aspects such as work quota in public projects, free or subsidised continual skill enhancement programs, subsidies for capital investment, incentives and commercial lending to micro and small sized organisations through a risk-sharing mechanism.

Methodological insights for researchers

This book demonstrated the application of a few advanced analytics techniques, namely classification and regression trees, cluster analysis and multidimensional scaling, for exploring work stress and its health consequences in construction. Drawing from the lessons learnt from this, the following insights are shared with other researchers in the construction management domain:

- Decision trees are a versatile, machine learning driven, analytics technique that can be used for tasks such as classification-based predictions, segmentation (grouping of objects), stratification (assigning cases to suitable categories), data reduction and variable screening (selecting significant predictors from a large set) and interaction analysis (identifying relationships). Moreover, they are easy to produce and can process non-normal data even in the presence of missing values. Yet, these are minimally used by construction researchers. Four statistical algorithms are widely utilised, namely: Classification and Regression Trees (CRT), Chi-squared Automatic Interaction Detection (CHAID), C5.0, and Quick, Unbiased, Efficient Statistical Tree (QUEST). This book demonstrated the application of CRT for analysing interactions among risk factors in producing various outcomes in two of the chapters. It further demonstrated how the results can be interpreted. These can be case studies and examples for other researchers who wish to apply the analytic technique in their research.
- Cluster analysis is a promising analytic technique that enables grouping of objects/cases by considering multiple data characteristics simultaneously and subsequently identifying the most significant data characteristics that are pertinent to an outcome. It identifies naturally occurring patterns in

datasets more effectively than traditional statistical techniques and can process non-normal datasets with missing values. Nonetheless, it is an underutilised technique by construction researchers. Three clustering techniques are available, namely non-hierarchical, hierarchical and two-step clustering. This book demonstrated the application of the two-step clustering technique twice for forming natural groups of outcomes based on the characteristics of over 20 predictors as well as for recognising the most influential predictors for the outcomes. These set examples for other researchers who may gain insights on the application of the technique and the interpretation of results.

- Multidimensional scaling (MDS) is a data visualisation technique that allows modelling and visually representing underlying/latent structures of relationships within a set of variables using perceptual maps. Despite its merits and wide use in many fields, MDS is an underutilised technique by construction researchers. This book demonstrated its methodical application and the interpretation of results, which can be a reference example and provide insights for other researchers.

Future research directions

Work stress is a relatively recent theme in the construction literature compared to other fields. Whilst it is possible to draw insight from studies conducted in other industry sectors, there are contextual factors that are specific to the construction industry, which make the manifestation of work stress and its consequences unique. Hence, pertinent studies are needed to explore the subject matter in context. Previous research has focussed on causes of work stress in the construction industry, particularly among while-collar professionals. This book extended this by investigating the consequences of work stress, specifically in the psychological and physical health domains. Yet, there are ample potentials for future research on work stress in construction. Some topics and themes are suggested for future research:

- This book established that work stress induced poor mental and physical health is quite widespread among construction professionals yet least discussed or not disclosed, possibly due to the fear of stigmatisation. The benefits of mobile computing can be utilised to pro-actively identify professionals who are experiencing chronic work stress and then commence early interventions. Future research may focus on developing a mobile app with a backend dashboard facility for regularly capturing psychosocial conditions experienced by employees in construction organisations. The data can be processed in the backend using suitable algorithms to produce work stress patterns, analytics and graphs on the dashboard. The mobile app itself should send queries/questionnaires regularly without the employee having to start the process of reporting. Since mobile apps are used for most things these days by almost everyone, this would be an easy strategy to practically implement.

- An Internet of Things (IoT) system may be developed for work stress management in construction organisations. The system could comprise two components, one for measuring the work stress levels in employees through signals from wearables and the other is a mobile relaxation app that is automatically triggered by the stress level measured by the wearable. The relaxation app may incorporate calming visual and audible contents such as funny sport scenes, comedies, magnificent nature images/3D virtual tours, and soothing sounds from nature – for example, birds, streams, rivers, etc. Moreover, the research may be extended to analyse the business benefits and the return on investment of the system.

- This book revealed that there is a lack of implementation of the three-tier stress interventions framework in construction organisations. Future research may be carried out to compute tangible business returns and benefits of implementing the framework in a bid to encourage organisations to implement it.

- Most of the research on work stress in construction focussed on white-collar professionals and only a limited amount of work can be found about operatives. Future research may be undertaken to investigate work stress among construction operatives, its causes and consequences in health and work performance domains.

- Studies of work stress in construction so far investigated the phenomenon in common for both genders. This book reveals that female professionals endure more work-related mental and physical strains. Though previous studies highlighted some key factors pertinent to females, dedicated explorations are required to understand the problem fully. Hence, future research may be undertaken separately to explore work stress among women professionals and women operatives in the construction industry.

- Most work stress studies in construction focussed on organisational and project-related causes for work stress. However, organisations exist in the wider market and the operations and work conditions of organisations are significantly influenced by the external factors. Future research is suggested to study work stress in construction from a holistic perspective with the use of the systems approach, contingency approach and/or socio-ecological approach as the overarching theoretical lens. For instance, the recent COVID-19 pandemic placed significant stress on organisations and individual employees. Similarly, government policies regarding capital investments as well as incentives and rebates for clients also impact on industry practices and market dynamics. There are several external factors that bear an influence on the operation of organisations. A holistic approach to work stress studies, covering individual, organisational, industry-wide, societal and governance aspects may be beneficial.

- In a similar systemic manner described earlier, future research is suggested to explore the challenges facing micro and small sized organisations in the construction industry, which eventually become risk factors for the deterioration of the physical and mental health of the proprietors of such organisations.

The research could also investigate viable and pertinent support mechanisms for the survival of this segment of the construction industry through different economic cycles and industry climates.

- This book demonstrated that time pressure or tight project schedules is a significant, recurring stressor and risk factor for several health and wellbeing concerns of construction professionals. Time pressure is often the cascaded effect of tight/unreasonable durations contracted for construction projects. Project durations are generally decided based on the cost and scope of the project. This is a deterministic approach. However, there may be various context specific factors that influence the productivity and progress and can result in various outcomes for two exactly similar projects. Some examples of such factors are procurement methods adopted, qualifications and experiences of the builder and subcontractors, disputes, completeness of project information and documentations and the timing/season of the start of construction. A stochastic model may be developed to help builders, design teams and/or clients determine optimum durations for construction projects, which would not compromise both the economic sustainability of the project and the social sustainability of the workforce that builds the project.

References

Parliament of Australia. (2019). Mental health in Australia: a quick guide. Retrieved 10 June, 2020, from www.aph.gov.au/About_Parliament/Parliamentary_Departments/Parliamentary_Library/pubs/rp/rp1819/Quick_Guides/MentalHealth.

Phillip, K. (2019). Six ways your office can reduce stress, 2019. Retrieved 20 July, 2019, from www.morganlovell.co.uk/knowledge/opinion-pieces/six-ways-your-office-can-reduce-stress/.

Appendix

Survey instrument

Consent/screening

As part of the requirement for ethical conduct of research, I am required to record your consent to participate in this survey. Your personal details are **not** required.

Do you consent to participate in the survey?
- ☐ Yes
- ☐ No

Are you 18 years or older?
- ☐ Yes
- ☐ No

Background information

The following questions concern your job role in general. No personal or organisational identity is required/collected. It is reminded that all questions are optional and only aggregated data will be reported.

1. Your gender:
   - ☐ Male
   - ☐ Female
   - ☐ Other

2. Please indicate your age range:
   - ☐ Below 20
   - ☐ 21–30
   - ☐ 31–40
   - ☐ 41–50
   - ☐ 51–60
   - ☐ Over 60

3. Your marital status:
   - ☐ Married/de-facto
   - ☐ Single, never married
   - ☐ Single, divorced/separated
   - ☐ Single, widowed

4. What is the main operation of your organisation?
   - ☐ Property developer
   - ☐ Project management consultancy
   - ☐ Architectural consultancy
   - ☐ Engineering consultancy (civil/structural/building services)
   - ☐ Cost management/Quantity surveying consultancy
   - ☐ Builder (Head contractor)
   - ☐ Subcontractor
   - ☐ Facilities management
   - ☐ Other (please specify):

5. How many people are working full-time in your organisation?
   - ☐ 4 or less employees
   - ☐ 5–19 employees
   - ☐ 20–199 employees
   - ☐ 200 or more employees

6. What is your job title? _____

7. How long have you worked in this role?
   - ☐ Less than 1 year
   - ☐ 1 to 5 years
   - ☐ 6 to 10 years
   - ☐ Over 10 years

8. Nature of your employment:
   - ☐ Permanent
   - ☐ Fixed-term contract
   - ☐ Casual

9. On average, how many hours a week do you work (including working from home office)?
   - ☐ Less than 20 hours
   - ☐ 20–30 hours
   - ☐ 30–40 hours
   - ☐ 40–50 hours
   - ☐ More than 50 hours

10. You predominantly work:
    - ☐ In an office environment
    - ☐ In a site environment

11. What is your annual income range?
    - ☐ Less than $40,000
    - ☐ $40,000–$60,000
    - ☐ $60,000–$80,000
    - ☐ $80,000–$100,000
    - ☐ $100,000–$120,000
    - ☐ $120,000–$150,000
    - ☐ Over $150,000

Job stressors

The following questions concern the presence of/exposure to stressors at work. It is reminded that all questions are optional and only aggregated data will be reported.

Reflecting the **past 6 months** in the current employment, please indicate how you assess the following statements about your job.

Job stressor	*Frequency*			
	Never	*Sometimes*	*Often*	*Always*
Job demand:				
1. You had to work in poor or dangerous physical work conditions	0	1	2	3
2. You had excessive workload	0	1	2	3
3. You had unpredictable work hours	0	1	2	3
4. You had excessive time pressure	0	1	2	3
Job control:				
5. You had a choice/say in deciding how you do your work	0	1	2	3
6. The work you performed was appropriate for your skills and abilities	0	1	2	3
7. You had flexibility with your work time	0	1	2	3
Support at work:				
8. You were given supportive feedback on the work you did	0	1	2	3
9. You could rely on your line manager to help you out with a work problem	0	1	2	3
10. If work got difficult, your colleagues helped you	0	1	2	3
Work relationships:				
11. You were subject to harassment in the form of unkind/unwanted words or behaviour at work	0	1	2	3
12. You were subject to bullying at work	0	1	2	3
13. You were subject to discrimination due to your gender, age or ethnic background	0	1	2	3
Role:				
14. You were clear what your duties and responsibilities were	0	1	2	3
15. You had enough resources to do your work	0	1	2	3
16. You were consulted on matters/changes that affected your job	0	1	2	3
Reward:				
17. Your salary was sufficient for the work you had to do	0	1	2	3
18. You had job security	0	1	2	3
19. You received rewards/appreciation for the efforts you put into your work	0	1	2	3
20. You had career progress opportunities	0	1	2	3

Work–private life conflict

The following questions concern the conflict between work and personal life. It is reminded that all questions are optional and only aggregated data will be reported

Over the **past 6 months**, how often did you experience the following work–private life conflict?

Indicator	*Frequency*			
	Never	*Sometimes*	*Often*	*Always*
1. Your work drained you so much of your energy that it had a negative effect on your private life	0	1	2	3
2. Your work took so much of your time that it had a negative effect on your private life	0	1	2	3
3. Your family or friends told you that you work too much	0	1	2	3
4. You encountered other personal life stressors on top of work stressors	0	1	2	3

Chronic job stress

The following questions concern whether you experience chronic job stress, whether diagnosed or not. It is reminded that all questions are optional and only aggregated data will be reported.

Over the **past 4 weeks**, how often did you experience the following chronic job stress symptoms?

Symptom	*Frequency*			
	Never	*Sometimes*	*Often*	*Always*
1. You slept badly and restlessly due to work issues	0	1	2	3
2. You had difficulty relaxing due to work issues	0	1	2	3
3. You were irritable due to work issues	0	1	2	3
4. You felt tense due to work issues	0	1	2	3
5. You felt nervous or anxious due to work issues	0	1	2	3

Stress coping methods

The following questions concern stress coping methods and strategies. It is reminded that all questions are optional and only aggregated data will be reported.

Over the **past 4 weeks**, how often have you engaged in the following activities to cope with work stress?

Stress coping method	Frequency			
	Not at all	*Several days*	*More than half the days*	*Nearly every day*
Positive / adaptive coping:				
1. Problem-solving (e.g. identified the source of stress and took an action to manage it)	0	1	2	3
2. Keeping a positive attitude (e.g. you looked for something good in what was happening in your life and tried to grow as a person as a result of the situation)	0	1	2	3
3. Seeking external support (e.g. you talked about the stressful event with a supportive person counsellor/friend/colleague)	0	1	2	3
4. Relaxation (e.g. you engaged in meditation, breathing exercises, sitting in nature, progressive muscle relaxation)	0	1	2	3
5. Physical activity (e.g. you engaged in team sports, exercise, yoga or swimming)	0	1	2	3
6. Engaged in humour, fun and leisure activities (e.g. gardening, movie, socialising)	0	1	2	3
7. Eating well-balanced meals	0	1	2	3
8. Resting and sleeping enough	0	1	2	3
Negative / maladaptive coping:				
9. Escape – isolating from others and making yourself busy with TV, reading, internet, etc.	0	1	2	3
10. Numbing – consuming alcohol or drugs to forget the stressful situation	0	1	2	3
11. Smoking to get a relief from stress	0	1	2	3
12. Emotional eating and drinking (eating comfort food and/or drinking coffee and other caffeine drinks to get relief from stress)	0	1	2	3
13. Criticising or blaming others for the situation	0	1	2	3
14. Compulsive spending – shopping and buying gifts for yourself to feel happy and forget stress	0	1	2	3
15. Ignoring as if nothing happened/try to forget the whole thing (denial/distancing)	0	1	2	3
16. Releasing tension by crying, yelling, throwing things, etc.	0	1	2	3

Physical and mental health effects

The following questions concern whether you experience health problems including physical and psychological ailments, whether diagnosed or not, due to work stress. It is reminded that all questions are optional and only aggregated data will be reported.

In the **past 6 months**, how often have you been bothered by/treated for any of the following health issues?

Health condition	How often have you been bothered by this illness?				Do you believe that job stress may have caused this illness?	
	Never	Once or twice	Monthly	Weekly	No	Yes
1. High blood pressure	0	1	2	3		
2. High cholesterol	0	1	2	3		
3. High blood sugar level	0	1	2	3		
4. Squeezing of the chest (angina)	0	1	2	3		
5. Heart muscle weakening	0	1	2	3		
6. Heart attack	0	1	2	3		
7. Stroke	0	1	2	3		
8. Diabetes	0	1	2	3		
9. Weight gain/obesity	0	1	2	3		
10. Gastrointestinal disorders	0	1	2	3		
11. Asthma	0	1	2	3		
12. Bronchitis	0	1	2	3		
13. Pneumonia	0	1	2	3		
14 Skin irritation/eczema	0	1	2	3		
15. Chronic headache or migraine	0	1	2	3		
16. Back, neck or shoulder pain	0	1	2	3		
17. Arthritis	0	1	2	3		
18. Blurred eye vision	0	1	2	3		
19. A weakened immune system/slower healing	0	1	2	3		
20. Sexual dysfunction	0	1	2	3		
21. Reproductive system disorder	0	1	2	3		
22. Insomnia	0	1	2	3		
23. Burnout	0	1	2	3		
24. Anxiety	0	1	2	3		
25. Depression	0	1	2	3		

Organisational interventions

The following questions concern organisational interventions that promote employee wellbeing. It is reminded that all questions are optional and only aggregated data will be reported.

Over the **past 6 months**, how often has your organisation applied the following interventions to promote wellbeing in the workplace?

Intervention	Frequency			
	Never	*Sometimes*	*Often*	*Always*
1. Implementing and/or improving polices and regulations on wellbeing and work conditions (workload, pay, career ladders, union involvement, work shifts, etc.)	0	1	2	3
2. Changing working conditions and/ or organisational practices for better wellbeing of employees	0	1	2	3
3. Training employees to improve skills or job roles	0	1	2	3
4. Training and educating supervisors and managers on wellbeing of subordinate staff	0	1	2	3
5. Training employees on stress management tactics				
6. Facilitating access to relaxation or exercise programs	0	1	2	3
7. Promoting peer support groups				
8. Providing psychological counselling/ therapy programs	0	1	2	3
9. Providing medical care and treatment for wellbeing issues	0	1	2	3
10. Providing rehabilitation and return-to- work programs for wellbeing issues	0	1	2	3

Job outcomes

The following questions concern adverse impacts of work stress on job outcomes. It is reminded that all questions are optional and only aggregated data will be reported.

Job satisfaction

On a scale from 0–10, where 0 is the *lowest* satisfaction anyone could have at your job and 10 is the *highest* job satisfaction, how would you rate your level of satisfaction with your current job in the past 6 months?

Lowest job satisfaction										*Highest job satisfaction*
0	1	2	3	4	5	6	7	8	9	10

Performance

On a scale from 0–10, where 0 is the *worst* performance anyone could have at your job and 10 is the performance of a top employee, how would you rate your *overall* job performance in the past 6 months?

Worst performance										*Best performance*
0	1	2	3	4	5	6	7	8	9	10

Acknowledgement

Thank you for completing the survey. We greatly appreciate your time. All responses and personal information will be confidential, held securely and remain unavailable to your employer.

Index

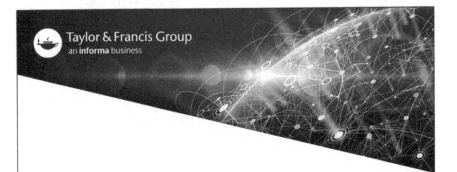

Printed in the United States
By Bookmasters